Comments on **Psoriasis – the 'at yo**
from readers

'Once again, I feel that this edition will be a gr[...]
with psoriasis, answering many of their questi[...]

Libby Pell, Community Dermatology Nurse,
Milton Keynes

'Being able to point people with psoriasis towards a book which will
help answer many of their questions in an easy and accessible format
has to be welcomed. The authors of this book clearly have great
experience of working through patients' concerns . . . given the
frequently disheartened stories we hear from the public about their
GPs knowing very little about Psoriasis, it should be required on every
medical school syllabus as well!'

Margaret Martin,
The Journal of the Psoriasis Association

'I am sure this book will be very well received.'

Dr Mary Judge, Consultant Dermatologist,
Royal Bolton Hospital

'I would recommend this book to all psoriasis patients and those
involved in their care. An informative, practice guide which will benefit
the individual with psoriasis and those providing specialist
dermatological care.'

Breege Fox,
British Journal of Dermatology Nursing

'An excellent and highly readable source of information for psoriasis
sufferers and their families. It gives you the facts and dispels many of
the myths.'

Ben Elton, Author and Comedian

'For those who may have just been diagnosed as having psoriasis,
this book will explain much about the disease, its symptoms and
treatments. It has medical remedies for keeping your skin in the best
possible condition, as well as exploring the psychological effects the
disease can have on the sufferer.'

John Bevan, Farnham

Comments on Psoriasis – the 'at your fingertips' guide from readers (continued)

'I would like to congratulate Dr Tim Mitchell and Rebecca Penzer on such an excellent book on psoriasis . . . it was a really good read. I am recommending it to all the people I know who suffer too.'

JC, Derbyshire

'Here it is: all you wanted to know but didn't like to ask your busy GP; all you were told but didn't quite grasp, or forgot as soon as you left the consulting room. Relax, and absorb the answers in comfort.'

Valerie Elliston, Colchester

'*Psoriasis – the "at your fingertips" guide* is an excellent resource and has pride of place on our desks at the Association. This second edition is very welcome and it is even more comprehensive. Everything you wanted to know about psoriasis is written in a clear and logical style. It answers those questions you forgot to ask your GP and it is full of suggestions to help you manage your psoriasis.'

Gladys Edwards, Chief Executive, Psoriasis Association

PSORIASIS

Dr Tim Mitchell MBCHB, DRCOG, DPD
*General Practitioner; Montpelier Health Centre in Bristol,
Founder Member of the Primary Care Dermatology Society;
Clinical Lead for Dermatology in Bristol North Primary Care Trust;
Adviser to the All Party Parliamentary Group on Skin*

Rebecca Penzer RGN, BSc(Hons)
PGDip Professional Education, MSc
*Independent Nurse Consultant, Opal Skin Solutions;
Trustee to the Psoriasis Association and the British
Skin Foundation; Member of the International Skin Care
Nursing Group Advisory Board*

CLASS PUBLISHING • LONDON

Printing history
First published 2000
Reprinted 2004
Second edition 2005
Reprinted with revisions 2007

The authors and publishers welcome feedback from the users of this book. Please contact the publishers.

**Class Publishing (London) Ltd,
Barb House, Barb Mews, London W6 7PA
Telephone: 020 7371 2119
Fax: 020 7371 2878 [International +4420]
Email: post@class.co.uk
Website: www.class.co.uk**

The information presented in this book is accurate and current to the best of the authors' knowledge. The authors and publisher, however, make no guarantee as to, and assume no responsibility for, the correctness, sufficiency or completeness of such information or recommendation. The reader is advised to consult a doctor regarding all aspects of individual health care.

A CIP catalogue record for this book is available from the British Library

ISBN 10: 1 85959 117 5
ISBN 13: 978 1 85959 117 8

10 9 8 7 6 5 4 3 2

Edited by Carrie Walker

Cartoons by Jane Taylor

Typeset by Martin Bristow

Printed and bound in Finland by WS Bookwell Juva

Contents

Acknowledgements

The authors particularly wish to thank the following individuals for their help during the writing of this book:

David Chandler, Psoriatic Arthropathy Alliance;
Gladys Edwards, Psoriasis Association;
Libby Pell, Milton Keynes PCT.

Foreword

by David Chandler

Co-founder, Psoriatic Arthropathy Alliance

Those of you reading this book who are newly diagnosed with psoriasis will quickly see that those burning questions that you felt were trivial, are echoed here. For people who have had psoriasis for a long time, this book may offer answers to questions that have long been puzzling you.

Finding uncomplicated, down-to-earth, common-sense advice is a valuable asset to living with a chronic disease such as psoriasis. As someone who has lived with psoriasis for more than 30 years, and psoriatic arthritis for almost as long, I have nearly forgotten the seemingly simple questions that needed answering when I was first diagnosed. This book would have answered those questions.

As a good, interesting read or as a quick reference when your psoriasis poses a problem at a particular time in your life, this book will educate you, help you to understand what is happening and how to cope, or guide you in asking further questions of your health-care givers.

This book will also enable those who live with or know someone who has psoriasis to gain an insight into why psoriasis is such a debilitating condition. The glossary and useful addresses add to the usefulness of this publication.

David Chandler

Introduction

Psoriasis is a chronic, recurrent inflammatory skin disease that affects 2–3% of the population in the UK. In simple terms, one person on a double-decker bus is likely to have the disease. Fair-skinned people, wherever they live, are equally affected by psoriasis, but it is much less common in African Caribbeans and Asians, and virtually non-existent in Inuit people and Native Americans. It affects men and women equally. The word 'psoriasis' comes from Greek words meaning 'the state of having the itch'. This reflects the fact that it has been around for many centuries, albeit being properly described only in the 20th century, and gives the lie to the suggestion in some medical textbooks that psoriasis does not itch. It also suggests that, although first described in the 1800s, psoriasis has been around for many centuries. It may well be that the Roman writer Pliny the Elder included psoriasis when he referred to disfiguring skin complaints that, although not painful or dangerous, were so distressing that 'any kind of death would be preferable'.

People's experience of itch can vary from none at all to severe; one in three people say that, for them, itch is the worst aspect of the condition. Other troublesome sensations, including burning, hurting and stinging, are also reported. Life can certainly be made miserable by the chronic itchy, scaly and inflamed 'plaques' that may occur on any part of the skin and scalp. A 'plaque' is the term for the scaly, red, raised patch of skin affected by psoriasis that can vary in size from 1 cm to 20 cm or more in diameter. People may find the condition disfiguring, and it can have a profound effect on their lives. We have some good examples of the misery of the disease in the writings of sufferers like John Updike and Dennis Potter, who had a severe form of psoriasis, but we must remember that the actual severity of the disease is not necessarily linked to its effect on the individual – seemingly trivial psoriasis can cause major psychological problems in some people, whereas others with what looks to be more severe psoriasis are able to cope better. It is vitally important that health professionals realise this, and that you, as someone with psoriasis, have a chance to talk about your feelings. Much of this book is devoted to the 'impact' of the disease on all aspects of life, and when we use the term 'management' we mean so much more than simply the treatments that are applied to the skin or taken by mouth.

It is worth noting here that the skin is, in fact, the largest organ in the body, with many important functions such as protection from the outside world, prevention of water loss and temperature regulation. These are in addition to the obvious cosmetic factor, where healthy skin and its ability to be decorated is of vital importance to the way we see ourselves and how others judge us on first impression.

Despite the potential impact of psoriasis, many people with this condition do not consult their doctors about it. One estimate indicated that up to 80% did not consult their GP over a period of a year. The reasons for this are probably many and varied, some people disregarding trivial psoriasis and others, with more severe disease, being despondent and fed up with the routine of applying messy creams day in, day out. Some may have had a less than sympathetic response from their GP. One reason for this response might be a lack of training in dermatology, resulting in GPs who are poorly equipped to deal with skin disease even though it can account for 15% of their workload. This omission is being tackled by various bodies such as the Royal College of General Practitioners, the British Association of Dermatologists and the Primary Care Dermatology Society, groups that represent GPs, consultant dermatologists and GPs with a special interest in dermatology, respectively. Additional support for better GP training has come from the All Party Parliamentary Group on Skin and various patient support groups, so it is to be hoped that the recently launched Core Curriculum in Dermatology for GPs in training will make an impact on patient care within the next few years. One problem is finding the time to fit in training on skin disease as GPs need to cover all aspects of medicine, but there are some proposed changes to the structure of the training programme that may make this easier.

In the meantime, favourite alternatives to consulting a GP include:

- no treatment at all;

- self-treatment;

- consulting practitioners of complementary therapies;

- holidays around the Dead Sea.

These alternative proposals are very understandable as, even with good-quality care, psoriasis can be a very stubborn condition to treat. It also has a remarkable and disheartening tendency to come back even after the skin has been clear for some time.

Many patients, and the public in general, are poorly informed about psoriasis. Misconceptions abound, causing upset, embarrassment and difficulty in accepting the various treatments. Commonly held beliefs include:

- it's infectious;

- it's an allergy;

- it's to do with the blood;

- it's *all* caused by stress;

- it will never get better.

None of these is correct. Moreover, psoriasis will get better and worse at times, regardless of the treatment being used. It can be difficult to explain why this happens, and it is very tempting to look at events preceding such change and see these as the cause. Thus, some people might believe that something like a change of diet made them better, but this would not apply to anyone else or even to that patient if their psoriasis worsened again. When psoriasis clears completely, either on its own or after treatment, doctors refer to it as being 'in remission', but the length of remission is very variable. This adds to the confusion about what has triggered an attack. What *is* clear is that there are a number of potential trigger factors, although the reaction will vary from person to person. Individuals will also respond differently to the same treatments, so whereas one person will find a treatment very helpful, another will find that it does not seem to work at all.

Psoriasis on its own can be a serious disease and more than enough for someone to cope with, but when it is complicated by such things as arthritis it can be very disabling. About 10% of people with psoriasis are thought to have arthritis as well, but the real number may be higher as not everyone will report it or link it to the psoriasis. Psoriatic arthropathy (arthritis) is common enough to have its own special name and is a particularly difficult form of arthritis that may – in one uncommon form – cause severe deformities of the joints in the hands. This can be quite disabling and, when combined with the skin disease, has a major effect on quality of life. Like psoriasis, the arthropathy has been around for thousands of years; the combination of swollen and twisted fingers with scaly skin matches some of the Biblical descriptions of lepers and probably resulted in people with psoriasis being shunned and even isolated from society in leper colonies. This attitude probably continued long after Biblical times as the disease itself was not properly described until the 19th century. To a certain extent, this isolation still occurs today, people with the condition being reluctant to use communal changing facilities, go shopping for clothes or even visit a hairdresser for fear of embarrassing stares or even being asked to leave because of others' ignorance about psoriasis. Children at school can have a particularly difficult time as teachers may insist that they do not take part in PE or swimming.

In today's National Health Service, there is great emphasis on informing and empowering patients, and this applies as much to people with long-term (chronic) skin problems such as psoriasis as to those with other diseases. All patients must have access to simple explanations about the disease, both verbal and on accessible, written information sheets. In addition, all patients who have just been diagnosed with psoriasis should be given the contact details of the relevant support groups. Every contact with a doctor should allow the chance for questions, however trivial the subject might seem – if it is worth asking, it is worth answering. This book is based on real questions asked by real patients, and we hope that we have provided some useful answers.

We also hope that the book will be read by people without psoriasis as well as those with it, and that it will serve as a way of increasing the awareness and understanding of this common disease. Much more public education is needed to allow for less prejudice towards sufferers – perhaps a few celebrities with psoriasis could admit to it when interviewed for glossy magazines!

Our background is in Western medicine, and we do not claim to have all the answers or that our approach is the only valid one, but we hope that our answers and comments will serve to provide hope and guidance to many of you. If only one reader decides that it is worth consulting a GP and demanding a better management of their skin problems, we will consider the effort of writing well worth it.

1
What is psoriasis?

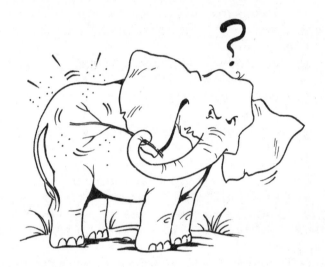

Introduction

Psoriasis is an inflammatory skin condition. The obvious sign is the colour change associated with the plaques (the raised patches on the skin), although this is more obvious where there is little scale. In fair-skinned people, the plaque will look red (sometimes referred to as salmon pink), whereas in dark-skinned individuals the plaque tends to look a darker shade of the normal skin. Often, however, the white scaling is thick and hides the redness, so psoriasis looks thick, white and crusty on exposed surfaces regardless of the underlying skin colour. The thickening is caused by the greatly increased 'turnover' of the skin cells. Normally, a living skin cell moves upwards from the bottom layer of skin, loses its nucleus and dies. It is then largely made up of a protein called keratin and is shed from the surface of the skin as new cells go through the same process and replace it from underneath. The whole process takes around 28 days, but in psoriasis it is greatly speeded up to a 3–4 day cycle. Living cells are then much closer to the surface, and as they still need a blood supply, the vessels lie closer to the surface, leading to the redness and heat that many people with psoriasis complain of. The fact that the surface cells are being replaced before they are shed results in a thick layer of scale, which, as everyone with the condition knows, flakes off readily and abundantly.

If you gently scratch the surface of a plaque, the scale starts to separate and looks silvery because it is not as tightly bound down as normal skin. Scratching harder removes the scale, with the appearance of multiple small bleeding points from the increased surface blood supply. Some parts of the body do not have this typical scale. These are usually the areas where two skin surfaces come together (occlusion), as in the natural skin creases and folds (e.g. the groin and genital region and the skin underneath women's breasts). In these areas, psoriasis can look bright red and shiny rather than scaly because the folds of skin come together, preventing evaporation and increasing the moisture content of the skin. The lesions do not dry out or scale as easily. This effect underlines the importance of applying lots of moisturising cream to plaques, as discussed later in the book.

The body's immune system plays an important part in this increased cell turnover as the altered genes in people with psoriasis seem to lead to a change in the function of a skin immune cell type, known as T-lymphocytes or T-cells. Lymphocytes make up the bulk of what are called 'white blood cells' and are probably best known for their role in dealing with infection. Their precise role in psoriasis has not been fully worked out, but they seem to be able to trigger the increased production of skin cells and attract other cells to the altered skin, which cause the inflammation. The importance of T-cells is borne out by the effect that some treatments that alter T-cell function have in psoriasis. This effect was discovered by accident when a transplant patient's psoriasis cleared up when he was given drugs to prevent rejection of his transplant. Such drugs block the production of T-cells and are discussed in Chapter 5. Further evidence for the importance of T-cells came from experience with patients receiving bone marrow transplants: specialised cells in bone marrow develop into T-cells, among others, and some patients who had received bone marrow from people with psoriasis developed the disease as they now had these 'abnormal' T-cells.

Because of this subtle way in which the immune system differs from normal, there may be some differences in the tendency for people with psoriasis to be affected by other diseases. This has some advantages as some diseases that might be thought of as 'allergic' are less common. Diseases that might be less common include atopic eczema, contact eczema and urticaria (hives). Some skin infections are also less common.

It is equally important to understand what psoriasis is *not*. This can be summarised by saying that it is:

- **not** contagious;
- **not** cancer;
- **not** related to diet; and
- **not** allergic.

A family connection?

There is psoriasis in my family but I am 40 and haven't got it. Does that mean I am lucky?

It might do, but some people seem to develop the disease later in life than others. There seem to be two peak times – one between the ages 20 and 30 and the other between 50 and 60. The first peak is much more likely to be associated with the 'psoriasis genes' and is starting to be called 'type 1' or 'early-onset' psoriasis. The later form tends to be less severe, is not usually associated with specific genes and is called 'type 2' or 'late-onset' psoriasis. There is obviously much more to be learnt about these different types, but you still have a chance of developing psoriasis.

My mother and I both have psoriasis. Is it hereditary?

Psoriasis can be described as a hereditary disease in that certain genes have been identified as being linked to psoriasis. These genes do not cause psoriasis but they make you more likely to develop it in response to certain 'triggers' that lead to the typical changes in the skin. Medical knowledge of the genes involved is increasing; two very important genes have been identified, along with several others that seem to play a minor role. This may help to explain the different patterns of psoriasis and the different responses to treatment discussed later in the book. Up to a third of people with the disease have someone in the family who has it as well, and having one particular gene on chromosome 6 (*Cw6*) makes it 24 times more likely that a person will get psoriasis. The other major gene is on chromosome 17.

Both my husband and I have psoriasis. Are the chances of our children getting it doubled?

The chances are much more than doubled, presumably owing to the chance of inheriting more than one of the 'psoriasis genes'. If only one of you had psoriasis, the chances of your children developing it would be only 15%; because both of you have it, the chance rises to 75%. It is always very difficult to answer individual questions about risk as the percentages are produced from studying large populations. If neither of you had psoriasis and your first child developed it, the chance of another child having it would be 20%.

Are eldest children most likely to get it?

No, all children will have an equal chance of inheriting the gene or genes involved, and there is no evidence to suggest that first-born children are more likely to be affected by the various factors that can trigger the disease.

I am pregnant; will my baby have my psoriasis?

Your baby will possibly have an increased risk of developing psoriasis if he or she inherits your 'psoriasis genes' but will not have 'picked it up' from you during the pregnancy even if your psoriasis has been bad. Because genetic material is passed on from both parents when an egg and sperm combine, your baby will only have a 50% chance of getting your genes and a 15% chance of getting psoriasis. This will apply equally to other children you might have.

If my children get psoriasis, will it be as bad as mine?

This is another question that is difficult to answer until we know much more about the different 'psoriasis genes' and their interplay with the various trigger factors. All we can say, really, is that nobody knows!

I didn't think there was any psoriasis in my family, but my 41-year-old sister has just developed it. What are my chances of getting it too?

It is not possible to give you a specific answer, because statistics only work for large groups of people. If you do develop the disease, you could look back and say that your risk was 100%, so any answer would be wrong! We hope, though, that you don't get it. You may be lucky because, although the overall risk in a case such as yours would be 20%, things are complicated by the age at which your sister developed the disease. Because she developed psoriasis after the age of 30, your risk is three times less than it would be if she had had it before the age of 15.

I have twin daughters but only one has psoriasis. Doesn't this suggest that it is not hereditary?

We can understand your confusion. Remember, though, that psoriasis is not caused by inheriting the suspect genes: they only make you more susceptible to the different triggers. Your daughter without psoriasis is lucky. Studies of large groups of twins help to show the hereditary basis: identical twins have a 65–70% chance of both developing psoriasis, but this falls to 15–20% for non-identical twins.

There is psoriasis in my family and I thought I had escaped, only to develop it after I was in a bad car accident. Why is this?

This is an example of a trigger factor switching on your inherited tendency to develop psoriasis. Certain things can trigger first or recurrent attacks of psoriasis, or just cause a flare-up of mild disease. These include trauma, infections, hormonal changes, some drugs and other serious illnesses. Good evidence for the importance of trigger factors comes from studying identical twins. Although both have the inherited tendency, there is only a 65–70% chance of both developing psoriasis. Different triggers are important for different people, which is why there can be difficulties in predicting and treating psoriasis.

Why have I contracted the disease when no one else in the family has it?

Although psoriasis is thought to be hereditary, it is really only the *tendency* to get the disease that is passed on in families. Some people can have an abnormal gene capable of causing psoriasis but it is never 'switched on', so the gene could have been passed to you from one of your (unaffected) parents. If not, it would mean that damage to the gene occurred during production of the sperm and egg that you developed from, or just after fertilisation. Before you develop psoriasis, some sort of trigger is needed; this could happen at any age as the disease can appear for the first time in infancy or old age.

Does psoriasis tend to skip a generation?

No, any pattern in a family suggesting this would have to be explained by looking at trigger factors. It is interesting, though, that there are several other diseases with a reputation for skipping a generation – for example, arthritis and diabetes.

Is it catching?

My husband has psoriasis ever so badly; will I catch it from him?

No. This is a commonly asked question and something that people are understandably concerned about. Psoriasis, like most other skin diseases, is not infectious or catching. People with psoriasis can get very upset by people who avoid touching them because they believe it is contagious, and this can increase the sense of embarrassment and isolation resulting from having different skin. It is very important that you do not 'shy away' from touching your husband, and he might especially value the contact if you help him to apply some of his treatments.

Psoriasis and other diseases

Does psoriasis ever turn to skin cancer?

No, there is no evidence that psoriasis is linked to skin cancer. One possible problem, however, arises from the treatment of psoriasis with ultraviolet light as this can contribute to the kind of skin damage that might turn into cancer if it is not strictly controlled. Many patients also find that their psoriasis improves in the sun, so they may expose themselves more and thus be more at risk of developing a skin cancer. This is explained further in Chapter 5, in the discussion of ultraviolet light treatment.

The scales on my scalp are yellow. Is this another type of psoriasis?

No. You probably have a condition called seborrhoeic eczema in your scalp, which is bad luck if you also have psoriasis elsewhere. Seborrhoeic eczema also causes redness and scaling on the scalp and can affect the face and upper body. On the scalp, there are several ways of telling one condition from the other. In seborrhoeic eczema, the scales are yellowish and greasy, rather than white and dry. If you pick the scales off, the skin underneath oozes clear fluid and blood all over in seborrhoeic eczema, but in psoriasis there are distinct points of bleeding. Seborrhoeic eczema is always itchy, but in psoriasis the itch varies from none to severe.

Can I get eczema as well as psoriasis?

Yes you can, but it is more likely to be the seborrhoeic form of eczema (mentioned above) than the 'atopic' form, which is the most common type in childhood. There may even be an overlap between seborrhoeic eczema and psoriasis as it can be very difficult to tell the two diseases apart, especially on the face. This may be quite a common problem, so some people use the term 'sebopsoriasis'. As we gain more understanding of the genetic basis of disease, we may reach a clearer understanding of why some diseases seem to 'overlap' – they may share some common gene patterns.

How can I tell eczema from psoriasis?

This can be difficult, especially when your hands, feet and scalp are involved or if the eczema is chronic, when it tends to be drier and thickened. Acute eczema tends to be more red, wet and weepy with no clear boundary between affected skin and normal skin. Psoriatic 'lesions' are thicker, with a silvery scale, and are well demarcated, i.e. it is obvious where the psoriasis stops and normal skin starts. This is equally true for the typical plaques and the bright red patches in the flexures (e.g. where the elbow and knee bend) and skin folds, where scale is not obvious. As with eczema, psoriasis tends to be symmetrical, which means that it tends to affect both sides of the body (e.g. both knees rather than just one). If you have scaly rashes that are not symmetrical, they may be due to some other cause, for example a fungal infection such as ringworm.

In older people, a first appearance of psoriasis tends to be more difficult to diagnose as it can look much more like eczema. Incidentally, their skin is also much more likely to be irritated by some of the common treatments, and this irritation can be much more like eczema.

My friend has been told that he has discoid eczema but it looks quite like my psoriasis.

Your confusion is understandable! Discoid eczema is a descriptive term given to a type of eczema that tends to present in the fourth or fifth decade of life. It favours the extensor surfaces of the limbs and, as the word 'discoid' suggests, takes the form of round lesions usually less than 5 cm across, which can be scaly or crusty. The scaling is not as white as in psoriasis, and it can sometimes be quite wet and oozing like an acute atopic eczema.

Is it true that some people with psoriasis are healthier otherwise?

As mentioned in the introduction to this chapter, the importance of the immune system in psoriasis does mean that some conditions may be more or less common in people with psoriasis. Those which may be more common are:

- chronic tonsillitis;
- obesity;
- raised blood pressure;
- heart problems;
- diabetes.

Those which may be less common are:

- atopic eczema;
- allergic asthma;
- urticaria;
- allergic contact eczema.

Overall, though, these possible differences in the chance of suffering from another disease are not great enough for our answer to your question to be anything other than 'No'.

Miscellaneous

Why is it thought that the immune system plays a part in causing psoriasis?

There are several reasons why the immune system is felt to be important in causing psoriasis. As discussed in Chapter 5, some immunosuppressive drugs (which damp down some parts of the body's immune reaction) work well in treating psoriasis. It is also a life-long disease, and this is taken as a sign that there is some 'memory' in the immune system that produces the typical rash of psoriasis in response to certain triggers. This 'memory' is part of the way our immune system works in recognising foreign bacteria and fighting them, and also explains why immunisation prevents us developing certain diseases. The way in which the disease can also clear up without treatment and then flare up again is also typical of a long-term immune response. One study has even shown that people who did not have psoriasis but had bone marrow transplants from someone with the condition went on to develop psoriasis. Finally, some of the genes identified are known to be linked to the way in which our immune system works.

Once clear, does psoriasis frequently recur?

Yes. Many patients will testify to this. One person we know has said that the worst thing about having psoriasis is that it 'always comes back'. It is difficult to be specific about individual cases as, once clear (in remission), it can stay away for a long time, but for most people it will recur all too often. About 50% of patients will have a spontaneous remission at some time, with perhaps 10% of them never having another attack. 'Spontaneous remission' means that a particular episode of psoriasis simply clears up on its own without any treatment.

My plaques feel especially hot. Why?

In psoriasis, the normal turnover time for the skin is greatly reduced. Normal skin will be replaced in around 28 days, with a slow cycle of new cells forming and turning to flat dead cells as they move up to the surface and are shed. In psoriatic skin, this whole process is speeded up to take only a few days. Less-mature cells are appearing on the surface of the skin, so the blood vessels that supply them are much closer to the surface than usual. Inflammation is also part of the psoriatic process, and this too leads to an opening up of the blood vessels. The skin feels hot because of the increased blood flow and, if the psoriasis is very extensive, this can be a serious problem because of the loss of body heat and fluid that evaporates from the hot skin surface. This is explained in Chapter 2.

2
Different types of psoriasis

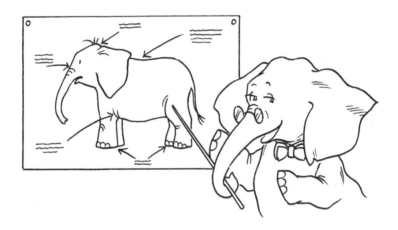

Introduction

As mentioned in Chapter 1, we now think that psoriasis is determined genetically, which means that people have an inherited tendency to develop the disease after certain triggers. Two main genes have been identified, with several other ones (perhaps up to 16 in total) playing a lesser part. The two main genes are called *PSORS1* and *PSORS2* and are found on chromosomes 6 and 17. This collection of different genes could explain why people can get different patterns of rash. The precise way in which the genes behave and interact has still to be worked out, and, as it is possible to inherit more than one of the genes, individual people may have more than one type of the disease, with varying degrees of severity.

Until all the genetics are fully worked out, we will have to rely on good descriptions of the patterns of psoriasis to identify the different types as this can affect the choice of the best treatment approach for each person.

One problem with the many different patterns of psoriasis is that some other conditions may be confused with it. These include eczema in its various forms; *seborrhoeic eczema* (mentioned in Chapter 1) is particularly confusing on the scalp. *Eczema on the hands and feet* can be difficult to tell from psoriasis, and even skin specialists (dermatologists) sometimes have to remove a piece of skin (under local anaesthetic) to be examined under a microscope – called 'doing a biopsy' – before they know exactly what label to give a rash! Another confusing pattern is *discoid eczema* (also mentioned in Chapter 1). As the name suggests, this occurs in little round areas a few centimetres across and can be quite thickened. It does not have the typical silvery scaling of psoriasis.

Other diseases that may cause confusion are ringworm and a condition called pityriasis rosea. *Ringworm* is more common in children and is usually itchy. It causes red patches on the body and often on the scalp. These patches can be a bit scaly and tend to grow outwards, leaving a clear area in the middle, so that they look like rings. The cause of ringworm is not a worm but a fungus, which also causes 'athlete's foot'. *Pityriasis rosea* is an odd-sounding name but just means 'bran-like' in Greek and 'pink' in Latin! It is a pink rash with fine scaling that appears only round the edge of each lesion and is thought to be a reaction to a viral infection. It first appears as a single patch 2–5 cm across, followed a week or so later by many more smaller oval patches on both sides of the body and upper arms. It can be confused with guttate psoriasis but clears up more quickly, often in about 6 weeks.

Types of psoriasis

What are the different kinds of psoriasis?

There are many different variations, which may be related to the belief that up to 16 genes can lead to a person developing psoriasis.

- **Guttate psoriasis** is also known as teardrop or raindrop psoriasis. It tends to occur in children, adolescents and younger adults, and is a generalised rash of small spots up to 1 cm in diameter. It tends to follow an infection, often of the throat, when it appears very suddenly a week or so after the infection. It is widespread but does spare the palms and soles, and clears up after several weeks or months depending on how quickly treatment is started. Up to 50% of people affected will not have a further attack, but the condition may become chronic or evolve into one of the other types of psoriasis.

- **Plaque psoriasis** is the 'typical' form with scaly red, raised patches – the plaques – which vary in size from a few millimetres to many centimetres across. They tend to be symmetrical and prefer the 'extensor' surfaces such as the backs of the elbows and the fronts of the knees. The lower back and sacral area (top of the buttocks) is another common site for large plaques. Although the plaques can be very large and widespread, they generally cover 5% or less of a person's body surface.

- **Flexural psoriasis** occurs in skin folds, in the armpits, under the breasts, in the groins and between the buttocks. It is described separately as the appearance is much less scaly, often being quite a bright, shiny red colour. In the groins, it can also affect the genitals. It can cause troublesome nappy rash in infants but is mainly found in older people. The reason for the lack of scale is the decreased water loss from two surfaces of skin lying against each other, so that the cells on the surface do not dry out, and this shows why applying a moisturising cream to psoriasis can be helpful in reducing scale, as discussed in Chapter 4.

- **Scalp psoriasis** is often very troublesome, with thick scale and redness that is also evident around the scalp margins. Nevertheless, the hair growth is not usually affected. Even if more hair falls out than normal or it seems to come away with the scale, it all grows back again.

- **Psoriasis on the face** is relatively uncommon and can be less clearly demarcated or scaly, leading to confusion with eczema.

- **Pustular psoriasis** can affect just the hands and feet, with yellow round pustules (raised areas of skin containing pus) appearing under the skin surface of the palms or soles, or both. They gradually turn brown as they reach the surface and are shed as scales. The pustules are sterile and not the result of infection. This pattern is most often seen in middle-aged people who are smokers. *Generalised pustular psoriasis*, with sheets of very small pustules on a background of very red, hot skin, is a medical emergency. A person can become very ill from loss of heat and fluid, and feel very feverish. It is sometimes triggered if large amounts of strong steroid creams have been used to treat widespread plaques or can occur after oral steroids given for any reason.

- **Erythrodermic psoriasis** is also an emergency. Like many medical terms, 'erythroderma' is from the Greek – for 'red' or 'inflamed' and 'skin'. The whole of the skin turns red and leads to a loss of fluid and heat, as with pustular psoriasis. There are no pustules, but urgent admission to hospital is needed to replace lost fluid and prevent hypothermia (low body temperature). Erythroderma can occur with other skin diseases such as eczema but is thankfully very rare. Whatever the cause, it looks the same, but in psoriasis, as with the pustular form, it can develop suddenly after the incorrect use or sudden withdrawal of steroid treatment.

- **Psoriasis of the nails.** There can often be changes to the nails. These range from discoloration and pitting of the surface to complete destruction of the nail. Psoriasis can make the nails split away from the nail bed and cause considerable thickening of the skin from under the nail. Severe nail changes can be very disabling and should never be dismissed as just being a 'cosmetic' problem.

- **Psoriatic arthropathy**. A final and very distressing type of psoriasis is that with arthritis. Psoriatic arthropathy may occur in up to 40% of people with psoriasis if X-rays are studied, but it may only be around 15% who have significant pain or disability. It can take several different forms, including one very difficult to distinguish from rheumatoid arthritis. Because arthritis itself is quite common, it can be difficult to decide exactly how many people with psoriasis truly have arthritis linked to their skin condition.

What is gutter psoriasis?

We think you mean guttate psoriasis. Guttate means 'drop-like' and is used to describe a type of psoriasis that is often the first manifestation in adolescents and young adults. It is an example of infection triggering the disease and often follows a sore throat, especially when a bacterium called *Streptococcus* is the cause. Very small, drop-like patches of psoriasis appear on the trunk and limbs, and may slowly clear on their own after several months. This can look quite dramatic, sometimes like having been splattered with red paint. Having an attack of guttate psoriasis does not necessarily mean that you will go on to develop other forms of the disease, but it may return if you suffer from the same type of infection again, so it is very important to see your GP quickly if you have had it before and feel another sore throat coming on.

Is there any way of preventing nails from pitting?

No. Pitting occurs when psoriasis affects the nail as it is formed. The tough horny layer forming the nail is weakened and partially collapses, forming pits 1 mm or less in diameter. They are usually randomly scattered on the nail and can affect both the fingernails and toenails.

I have psoriasis in my ears. Will I go deaf?

The ear canals leading from the outside to the eardrum are simply rolled up tubes of skin, so psoriasis can occur there. It will not cause permanent deafness from damage to the ears, but it can lead to the canal being blocked with scales and wax, muffling the hearing. Treatment can be difficult, and you might need to have your ears cleaned out at the ear, nose and throat (ENT) department of your local hospital. Do not be tempted to try to clean out the ears with cotton buds as this can compact the debris at the end of the canal and make the problem far worse.

Can I get psoriasis in my mouth?

It is possible to get psoriasis in the mouth as it can affect the mucous membranes – the term for the lining of internal surfaces such as the mouth and gut. This is quite rare, though, and tends to occur only with severe psoriasis, especially the pustular type (explained on page 15). There is a weak link between psoriasis and a condition called 'geographic tongue', in which the surface of the tongue varies in texture and colour from loss of the normal roughness to increased reddening of the smoother areas. It can look like the outline on a map, hence its name.

Psoriatic arthropathy

What is psoriatic arthropathy?

As if it were not enough to have psoriasis, some people have the added problem of a form of arthritis specific to psoriasis – called psoriatic arthropathy. This is probably much more common than previously thought as one study that examined people with psoriasis and took X-rays of their joints showed changes recognised as being due to arthropathy in half of them. Most of these people had absolutely no symptoms, so the percentage of people who really suffer from the condition is closer to 15%. It can be wrongly diagnosed as being due to other causes of arthritis, especially as it can occur before there are any signs of psoriasis on the skin. The arthritis can affect one or more joints as well as the bones in the spine and can cause painful local swelling and stiffness. One form can be quite destructive to the joint, causing severe disability.

Are there different types of arthritis as mine is different from a friend's and we both have psoriasis?

Psoriatic arthropathy can be classified into five different types, so the answer is 'Yes'! Although it is easy to write down the differences between these different types, things are not so clear-cut in real life as one person may have features that fit several types, and there is progression from one type to another.

- The most common presentation is probably with swelling of one or two large joints on one side of the body. This is called asymmetrical oligoarthritis and accounts for 70% of cases. It often progresses to affect more joints on both sides of the body – referred to as symmetrical polyarthritis.

- Symmetrical polyarthritis is thought to make up 15% of cases and is the type that most closely resembles rheumatoid arthritis. The blood test that is positive in rheumatoid arthritis will be negative here, however. The condition affects many joints at the same time and can be found in both large and small joints. This can be a very troublesome form of the disease as about half of people with this type will experience slow worsening with more and more damage to their joints.

- Another pattern just picks out the small joints in the fingers, especially where there are nail changes as well.

- The spine can also be affected, as can the parts of the body where large tendons join strong muscles on to bone, for example the Achilles tendon where it attaches to the heel, and around the pelvis. This leads to pain and stiffness, which is particularly bad in the lower back.

- Finally, one form of arthropathy is very destructive – hence the name 'arthritis mutilans'. It is very severe and affects the small joints of the hands as well as the feet and spine. The joint destruction can leads to loss of use and great disability.

The last three types are thought to make up 5% each of the overall problem of arthropathy.

With psoriatic arthropathy, does the psoriasis rash on the skin appear at the same time as the arthritis?

It can do, but it can also appear before and after. The majority of people (60%) will have the rash before the arthropathy, 15% will get both at the same time, and 25% will get the joint problems first. If you get the arthropathy first, it can be very difficult to identify the cause, so your doctor will want to look at your nails for any early changes, such as pitting, and to ask whether anyone in your family has psoriasis.

Do men and women stand an equal chance of getting arthropathy?

Overall, yes, but there are some interesting differences in the chance of getting one type or another that does not yet have any explanation. Men are more likely to get the types that affect the hands and the spine, and women are more likely to suffer from the symmetrical polyarthropathy that looks like rheumatoid arthritis.

My fingers have swollen up. I have read that you can have arthritis with psoriasis – could this be my problem?

You could have one of the types of arthritis linked with psoriasis: it depends on where the swelling appears. If it just affects the last joints of your fingers, perhaps where you have some nail changes, and is not the same on both sides, it is likely to be the type that just affects these small joints and is unlikely to get very much worse. If, however, the fingers as a whole swell up, with pain in the knuckles and an even pattern in both hands, it could be the more generalised and troublesome form of the disease that can be confused with rheumatoid arthritis. You should seek help from your doctor quickly. Swollen fingers are sometimes called 'sausage fingers' because of their appearance. A medical term is 'dactylitis'.

The swelling of arthropathy is usually accompanied by pain, tenderness and stiffness. If you don't have any of these other problems, you might have swelling from another cause, such as infection or fluid retention, which would need completely different treatment.

Is there a blood test I can have for the arthritis associated with my psoriasis?

No, there isn't. It would be much simpler if there were a test, but this type of arthritis is called 'sero-negative' because nothing shows up when the serum part of the blood is tested. It is important, though, to do this test if the arthritis is symmetrical as it can be confused with rheumatoid arthritis, which is usually 'sero-positive' – more than 80% of people with this disease have a substance called rheumatoid factor in their blood.

A test you might be offered looks at levels of inflammation in your body and can be very useful in determining whether or not your arthritis is very active – this can help with deciding to have different types of treatment. It can look at the 'ESR' (the erythrocyte sedimentation rate – the speed at which the red blood cells settle under gravity in a tube) or the 'viscosity' (stickiness of your blood). Both of these would be raised if you had a lot of inflammation.

These tests are not helpful in deciding whether or not you have psoriatic arthropathy, because they indicate inflammation from any cause, such as severe infection or some diseases that cause inflammation in the gut.

Is it possible for me to have arthritis that is not caused by my psoriasis?

Yes, indeed. Just because you have psoriasis, it does not mean that any aches and pains should be labelled as being due to psoriatic arthropathy. You are just as likely as people without psoriasis to have osteoarthritis or rheumatoid arthritis, or even conditions such as gout that can be confused with the type of psoriatic arthropathy that only affects one joint. Only 4% of people with generalised arthritis have the psoriatic form. Although the early treatment of painful joints may be much the same whatever the cause, it is important for you to discuss things with your GP and make sure you are having any appropriate tests. There are developments in imaging techniques using MRI (magnetic resonance imaging) scanners that might make it easy to diagnose psoriatic arthropathy in the future.

Is it just an added nuisance to have the joint problems or is it more serious if you do?

It can be a serious problem as there is an increased mortality (chance of dying) if you have very bad arthropathy, i.e. if your ESR or blood viscosity is raised, showing a high level of inflammation, and you have X-ray changes around the joints. The powerful treatments used in severe cases also carry a risk.

I have only a little bit of psoriasis but have some painful joints. Isn't it just people with lots of psoriasis who get the arthritis?

No, unfortunately anyone with psoriasis can get joint problems – sometimes before they know they have the skin disease. People with severe psoriasis are, however, more likely than others to get arthritis – perhaps 25% of them will suffer compared with 15% for all people with psoriasis. As you have found out, though, this difference is irrelevant at an individual level.

Cause or effect?

Sometimes I pick off the top layer of scaly plaque. Does this damage my skin in any way?

It will not lead to permanent direct damage, but it can cause problems because the skin will bleed very easily under the scale and you could introduce infection. Plaques do tend to get very itchy as they dry out, and many patients do scratch or, like you, try to pick off the scales to stop the itch. It would be much better to smooth on a moisturising cream or ointment. If you did more than just picking off the scales and really damaged the underlying skin, you would encourage more psoriasis to develop.

I recently had my appendix out and now have psoriasis in the scar – why is this?

This is an example of a very common and troublesome problem for people with psoriasis. The disease can occur after any damage to the skin such as a wound or even a bad scratch. This is called the Koebner phenomenon after a German dermatologist who described the reaction in the 19th century. It also occurs with other skin problems such as warts.

How can I stop the irritation?

The best way to stop the irritation is, of course, to treat the psoriasis so that it clears up. This is often easier said than done, but simply moisturising the skin with a greasy preparation can help greatly. It will also prevent the plaques from drying out and cracking, which can make them very sore – a common problem in cold, dry weather. It is also helpful to keep yourself cool. Try to avoid getting hot and sweaty as we have found that these are the times when psoriasis gets most itchy.

When the psoriasis falls from my scalp, is it 'dead skin'? I have found that when a piece falls on to a part of my body, it irritates and makes me scratch, and a patch appears later. Am I imagining this or is the psoriasis still alive?

The scale falling from your scalp is dead and cannot cause psoriasis anywhere else. Even a living cell picked out from a patch of psoriasis would not affect any other part of the skin as psoriasis is not infective and cannot be caught. The scale falling on your skin creates a sensation, which you may interpret as itch. It is the resulting scratching that can give rise to a patch of psoriasis in your skin as it already has the potential to develop the disease. This is an example of the 'Koebner phenomenon' mentioned above.

Wherever I go, I leave a snowstorm of scales behind me. How can I reduce this?

This is such a common and difficult problem for people with psoriasis. You must find it very restrictive and embarrassing. Leaving snowstorms can make it very difficult to stay in other people's houses and to do everyday things such as wearing dark clothes or trying on clothes in shops. As with irritation, it can be helped by using a moisturiser frequently throughout the day. Some people notice that their psoriasis dries up and sheds more scale as it starts to get better, welcoming this as a good sign.

3

What triggers psoriasis and what makes it worse?

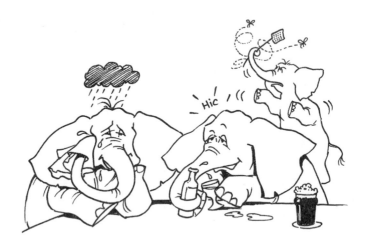

Introduction

As mentioned earlier in this book, genetic changes can give you the tendency to develop psoriasis, but some trigger is needed to start the process off. A variety of trigger factors have been identified, but more research is needed, especially into why some areas of the skin will develop psoriatic plaques whereas other areas remain normal. It can be very difficult to make generalisations from what we call 'anecdotal evidence' of individual patients' beliefs about triggers, but the following list reflects those events or things which do seem able to have an effect on all patients with psoriasis at some time:

- stress and emotional upset;
- infection;
- injury to the skin – even a simple scratch or insect bite;
- puberty, menopause and pregnancy (changes in hormone levels);
- some prescribed drugs (e.g. beta-blockers, chloroquine and lithium);
- alcohol in excess;
- smoking;
- poor general health;
- changes in climate;
- severe damage to the immune system (e.g. with AIDS or after chemotherapy for cancer);
- exposure to ultraviolet light (rarely).

Diet

Does diet affect psoriasis?

There is little scientific evidence that suggests a direct link between diet and psoriasis. It is wise for everyone to have a healthy balanced diet that contains lots of fresh fruit and vegetables (at least five portions per day), and to drink plenty of fluids (1.5–2 litres a day), especially water. Following these sensible guidelines will help you to stay healthy, which will have a beneficial effect on your skin. It is worth saying that some people feel very strongly that certain foods, for example tomatoes, do make their skin feel worse. If you think this is the case and you feel you can identify which foods worsen your skin, it is worth avoiding them. It may be that you have an additional problem called urticaria (or hives), which can be triggered by some foods, and you should discuss this further with your GP. Urticaria is not related to psoriasis and has other causes as well as reactions to some foods.

When I drink a lot of alcohol my skin feels worse the next day. Why is this?

Alcohol has the effect of dehydrating the body (i.e. removing excessive amounts of water), which is one reason why a headache is part of a hangover. This dehydration also affects the skin and causes it to become drier. Consequently, if you have had excessive amounts of alcohol, you are likely to make your psoriasis drier – which will make it feel worse. Having one or two alcoholic drinks in an evening should not have an adverse effect, but drinking enough to get drunk or having more than 10 units in one evening may make your skin worse.

People sometimes find themselves drinking excessive alcohol as a way of coping with their psoriasis. This is not a helpful coping strategy and, as highlighted here, will actually make your skin worse. Some of the treatments for severe psoriasis (e.g. methotrexate – discussed in Chapter 5) make it dangerous to drink alcohol. Methotrexate is broken down in the liver, as is alcohol. Drinking alcohol while taking methotrexate can put an extra strain on the liver and may damage it.

There is some evidence that alcohol can be involved in triggering psoriasis rather than just making it worse – a suggestion that is denied by many patients. We have been told by some patients that if we had psoriasis, we would drink too! If you feel your alcohol consumption is becoming a problem, you should discuss this with your doctor.

Stress

Is psoriasis affected by rest or stress?

There is increasingly good scientific evidence to suggest that stress has an important role to play in developing psoriasis. It is helpful to consider two extreme points of view. For some people, there is a very clear relationship between stressful events and their psoriasis flaring up. This connection is so direct that they can feel the psoriasis getting worse or throbbing when they are in a difficult situation. Other people cannot find any direct relationship between experiencing stressful events and their psoriasis flaring up. The simple answer, then, is that stress can make psoriasis worse, and for most people the role that stress plays is somewhere between the two examples given here.

It is sometimes difficult to identify the stressful event that makes psoriasis worse; it may be that a period of time passes between a stressful event and the psoriasis worsening. The other issue that is very clear is that having psoriasis itself is a stress. Thus, getting a flare-up of psoriasis may set off a vicious circle whereby the flare-up causes stress that makes the psoriasis worse, which causes stress . . . Effective and timely treatments are of particular importance as they help to break the vicious circle or even stop it from starting in the first place.

Rest is important, and finding time to unwind from a busy work or home life helps to keep stress under control. Simple things like having enough sleep help to increase your resilience and decrease the effect of a stressful lifestyle. A rest from the seemingly endless routine of applying creams to your skin can also help greatly. It may be possible for you to get support doing this from nurses in your local dermatology department or nurses at your GP practice. Alternatively, having a friend or relative who can help you is invaluable.

If psoriasis is stress related, what can be done to reduce stress levels?

This is a difficult question to answer as everyone is different in terms of what helps them to reduce stress. There are, however, a number of strategies that it is useful to consider.

First of all, you can identify the things that cause you most stress in your life and consider whether it is possible to change or avoid these. It may be useful to sit down and talk about these with someone close to you or with your own nurse/doctor. It is sometimes difficult to do this task alone because you are so close to the stress factors that it is hard to recognise them. If you cannot remove or change the things that cause you stress (e.g. it may not be possible to change your job or get rid of your kids!), you need to use strategies that help you to relax and create time for yourself. This is where individual preference comes in. For some people, playing sport might provide a therapeutic outlet for stress. For others, having a massage, trying reflexology or starting meditation may provide the answer. The underlying message of this advice is to create space and time for yourself to allow you to do something that makes you feel good. The temptation may be to indulge in something that makes you feel good in the short term but has no real long-term benefits, for example heavy drinking. This sort of destructive activity is known as a negative coping strategy and, rather than helping the situation, will probably make it worse.

The second thing that can be done to reduce stress levels is to get effective treatment. Psoriasis and stress tend to be a vicious circle – stress can trigger psoriasis, which, when it appears, makes you feel more stressed, which makes your psoriasis worse and so on. Getting treatment that makes your skin feel and look better and that fits in with your lifestyle can break the vicious circle.

To summarise, you need a two-pronged plan to remedy the impact of stress: first, a mental approach that helps you to relax more and create time for yourself; and second, a physical approach which ensures that your psoriasis has a minimal physical impact.

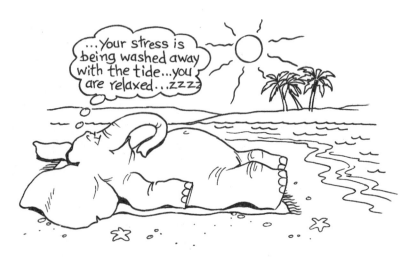

Other triggers of flare-ups

What usually makes psoriasis flare up?

As mentioned in the answer above, stressful lifestyles and specific stressful events are thought to be a possible cause, or 'trigger', of flare-ups.

Certain drugs are known to aggravate psoriasis; these include the antimalarial drug chloroquine, the antidepressant lithium, and anti-arrhythmic drugs and beta-blockers, usually used to treat heart disease or high blood pressure. If you are taking any of these drugs, it may be that you cannot discontinue them, and you should certainly not do so without consulting your doctor. It is, however, worth discussing this with your doctor as there may be alternatives that do not have a triggering effect. The problem with chloroquine is worth remembering, especially if you are planning a holiday to improve your psoriasis: it would be a shame to make it worse by taking chloroquine. Although you must not ignore the need to take antimalarial drugs if you are holidaying in an area where malaria is present, there are alternative antimalarial drugs that will not make psoriasis worse.

A throat infection, especially a 'strep' sore throat (caused by the *Streptococcus* bacterium) can trigger guttate psoriasis. (See also the next question and Chapters 1 and 2 for further details.)

Damaging the skin (e.g. a cut from falling over or from surgery) can trigger psoriasis at the point of the injury. This is known as the Koebner phenomenon (see Chapter 2 as well). The skin does not have to be broken for this to occur. Many of you will be familiar with the fact that psoriasis develops where your clothes rub (e.g. round the belt line); this too is the Koebner phenomenon, caused by the constant rubbing of material against the skin. Scratching itchy patches of psoriasis may also aggravate the psoriasis because scratching can damage the skin.

For most people, sunshine is very helpful in improving the psoriasis, but for about 10% of people with psoriasis, sunlight actually makes the condition worse.

My doctor says I have got it because of a sore throat.

Guttate psoriasis, a specific type of psoriasis in which a lot of small raindrop-like spots appear across the body, is often triggered by a streptococcal throat infection. It is this infection which gives you the sore throat. Your doctor may advise you to see him or her whenever you have a sore throat so that you can be treated with antibiotics. This may stop the psoriasis developing.

Can an infection cause psoriasis to flare up?

As mentioned in the previous answer, a streptococcal infection can lead to a flare-up of guttate psoriasis. Other sorts of infection may aggravate psoriasis in that they make you feel generally more run down and thus more susceptible to the stresses of everyday life. There is, however, not the same direct connection that there is between the streptococcal infection and guttate psoriasis.

What about serious infections like HIV?

HIV infection can make psoriasis and psoriatic arthropathy worse. This is in contrast to the effect that the virus has on rheumatoid arthritis, which can get better after HIV infection.

My psoriasis is always better in the winter than in the summer, but my cousin's is better in the summer. Why is this?

It is fair to say that your cousin's situation is more usual than your own. Most people find that, as soon as they are able to expose their skin to the sunshine in summer, their psoriasis shows some signs of improvement. For many people, the cold, dark winter months make their skin worse. It may be that you are one of the few people (about 10%) for whom sunshine makes the skin worse, which is why your skin is better in winter than summer.

Does biological washing powder make it worse?

Unlike eczema, psoriasis does not tend to be sensitive to external 'sensitisers' – irritants that cause the skin to become inflamed. So the simple answer is that it is very unlikely. However, if you were sensitive to washing powder anyway or had an irritant reaction to an ingredient that meant that your skin was damaged (either through the rash or through you scratching), psoriasis might develop because of the Koebner phenomenon (see earlier in this chapter).

Is psoriasis linked to fungal changes?

Having a fungal infection – athlete's foot or ringworm – does not cause psoriasis, but some types of fungus may infect nails damaged by psoriasis. Some of the nail changes in psoriasis and fungal infection can look very similar, so it is worth checking this out, especially if only a few nails are affected. Your GP should be able to arrange for nail clippings to be examined for evidence of fungal infection. Some fungal infections on the skin can look very like small patches of psoriasis with redness and scale.

Is psoriasis linked to hormonal fluctuations?

Some women report that their psoriasis seems to vary according to their monthly cycle, but there is no clear scientific evidence for this. Likewise, most women find that their psoriasis improves during pregnancy, only to return once they have given birth. The reverse is, however, also true as other women find that their psoriasis gets worse during pregnancy. In women, psoriasis often starts at puberty or the menopause, which does suggest that the changes in hormone levels may trigger psoriasis.

It might seem logical to think that, if hormonal changes apparently trigger psoriasis, a possible treatment would be hormone therapy. Unfortunately, the link between the hormonal changes and developing psoriasis is not that straightforward, and hormone treatment is not being seriously investigated at present.

4
First-line treatments

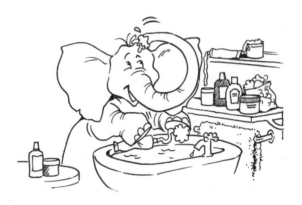

Introduction

Because psoriasis can come and go over a lifetime, it is important that people with the disease feel empowered to manage it themselves. This means that they should be as well informed as possible and feel confident that their own views are listened to when decisions about treatments are taken. Health-care professionals should provide help, education, support and treatment advice when necessary. They should also put you in touch with the relevant support group – there may even be a local support group that you can contact. Treating psoriasis should be a team effort, the team members varying according to the needs of the person concerned. Treatments need to be acceptable to the individual as well as being effective, so it is important that health-care professionals understand your view of the disease. The cost of treatment in terms of both time and money has to be taken into account, and the chore of applying creams once or twice a day can dampen one's motivation to treat the skin over a prolonged period.

It is, therefore, very important to avoid looking at the psoriasis on its own because treatment is much more likely to succeed if it is firmly grounded in the context of your life, beliefs and needs for treatment. Expectations, especially unrealistic ones, must be explored and discussed.

'First-line treatments' are the initial treatments that your doctor or nurse will suggest to manage your psoriasis. These are topical, i.e. applied directly to the skin. For mild-to-moderate psoriasis, they are usually all that are required to control it successfully. If your psoriasis is severe and/or does not respond to first-line treatments, your doctor may recommend a move to second-line treatments (discussed in the next chapter). Overall, some 75% of people with psoriasis need no more than these topical treatments, and one of the main reasons for failure seems to be a lack of ability or willingness to continue with the treatment according to the instructions. This used to be called a lack of 'compliance' with treatment but is now referred to as a lack of 'concordance' – which means agreement and reflects the input that you, the person with psoriasis, must have into the choice of treatment.

First-line treatments generally involve applying creams and ointments to the skin (topical treatment); when used properly, they have minimal side (unwanted) effects. There are lots of different treatments on the market, often with a bewildering variety of names, and many manufacturers make extravagant claims about their success. However, the fundamental components of first-line treatments usually belong to a fairly limited list.

Whatever treatment you use, **moisturisers** will be the mainstay. Moisturisers are substances used to moisturise the skin, either by being rubbed in or by being put in the bath or shower. They are also good to use instead of soap as the detergents in soap can have a very drying effect on the skin. There is a huge range available, and every individual should be able to find an acceptable one. More descriptions of and explanations for the use of moisturisers are given later in this chapter. Moisturisers are sometimes known as emollients – in effect they are two words used to describe the same thing.

Tar is a useful substance to treat psoriasis, although it tends to have a strong smell and can be very messy. Tar-based products range from weak substances (e.g. in Exorex) to much stronger ones (e.g. coal tar and salicylic acid, which tends to be prepared and used in hospital departments). Although there is no conclusive evidence linking the use of coal tar with cancer, there have been concerns about the risk in people who use it extensively over long periods of time. Tar can be used on small or large plaques of psoriasis, and although it can irritate unaffected skin, this is only transient and mild, and makes tar suitable for psoriasis that does not have a definite edge and/or is widespread across the body. Tar is not generally recommended for delicate areas of skin (e.g. skin folds or the face), but it can be very useful for pustular psoriasis on the hands and feet.

Dithranol, now manufactured chemically, was originally produced as an extract from a special tree bark. Its value in psoriasis was discovered by accident when a patient with psoriasis and arthritis was given a powder produced from the tree to treat the arthritis. His psoriasis cleared even though the arthritis did not. Dithranol is now used to treat well-defined plaques of psoriasis. It can irritate quite seriously if it is allowed to get on to skin with no psoriasis on it, so it needs to be applied carefully. It is usually applied for a short period of time before being washed off. Dithranol does not smell, but it does tend to stain clothes and surrounding furniture a distinctive purple colour.

Vitamin D derivatives, for example Dovonex (calcipotriol), Curatoderm (tacalcitol) and Silkis (calcitriol), are newer treatments for psoriasis and have the advantage of being relatively clean and non-smelly. They are easy to apply, and although some people have experienced a degree of irritation, this is usually fairly mild and only temporary. Calcipotriol is now available combined with a potent topical steroid in a formulation called Dovobet; this is particularly useful for treating inflamed psoriasis but should not be used for more than 4 weeks without being reviewed by a doctor.

Vitamin A derivatives, for example Zorac (tazarotene), are also relatively new to the list of available topical treatments. They are applied only once a day and can be used for up to 12 weeks. Zorac comes in gel form and is relatively clean and non-smelly, but it can cause irritation on the face and in skin folds.

Topical steroids are not routinely used for treating chronic plaque psoriasis because, although potent or very potent steroids can have a very spectacular positive effect, the psoriasis often comes back (rebounds) as badly if not worse than before once they have been stopped. The short-term use of steroids can, however, be very helpful, especially when psoriasis is inflamed or when it exists in delicate areas of the skin (e.g. the skin folds or face). They are also used in combination with other treatments, and one preparation (Dovobet; see above) contains calcipotriol and a potent steroid – this is licensed for use of up to 6 weeks, although it should ideally be reviewed at 4 weeks.

One other type of drug is starting to be used by specialists for topical treatment and may become available for GPs. It is called Protopic (tacrolimus) and is an immunomodulator that was designed for the treatment of atopic eczema. It has proved promising for treating psoriasis where the plaques are quite thin and without scale – such as in those delicate and sensitive areas mentioned above.

Topical treatments often take 4–8 weeks to have any effect, which can be quite demoralising. They can, however, work very well, and the best strategy is to choose treatments that fit best into your lifestyle. It is very important that you use the correct amount of any cream or ointment: some treatments need to be applied sparingly, whereas others are put on more thickly. Many people notice that if one of two plaques start to fade with the treatment, others do so of their own accord. If treating all the psoriasis seems too much trouble, it is worth tackling the bits that are most bothersome and seeing whether the others fade by themselves. We would always recommend that you put moisturiser on all over your body as this really does help to soothe and smooth.

What sort of treatment?

How does my doctor decide which treatment is most suitable for me?

The doctor will make the decisions about what treatments are most suitable for you based on three main factors:

- The extent and location of your psoriasis will be a major

consideration. Some treatments are suitable for mild-to-moderate psoriasis but are not as helpful for severe psoriasis. Similarly, some treatments are suitable for your trunk, arms and legs but not for your face.

- Your lifestyle should also influence what your doctor prescribes. He or she should check with you on issues such as how much time you have to give to doing treatments, whether you have a partner who can help you and what sort of job you do. These are important because, whatever treatment you are prescribed, you have to be willing and able to use it – treatments do not help psoriasis if they stay in their pots!

- It is also important that you and your doctor both have the same idea about what treatment success means. You might want your skin to be completely clear, or you may be very happy if it does not itch and there is no psoriasis visible when wearing normal clothes. Make this clear and you are more likely to be pleased with the results.

When I apply the creams to treat my psoriasis, what should I expect to see by way of improvement?

There are a number of changes that you should see if you are using the treatments properly and often enough. Applying moisturisers regularly will make your plaques less scaly, less itchy, softer and more flexible. They will not make the plaques any smaller, but they will make it easier for the other treatments to get through the thickened skin and do their job. Whichever type of 'active' treatment you are using (e.g. tar, dithranol or vitamin D creams), you will notice that the psoriasis tends to clear from the centre of the plaque outwards. The plaques themselves will not shrink in size, but clear areas of skin will appear in the centre of the plaques, leaving outer rings that will be the last bits to clear up. You can also tell by touch that the centre is clear by running your finger over it and feeling how smooth it is. Dithranol, uniquely, temporarily stains the skin a purple/brown colour. This staining occurs only on skin cleared of psoriasis, so you know when the psoriasis has gone because your skin turns purple! The stain will disappear completely in a couple of weeks.

How long does it take for the plaques to disappear when I use the creams?

The length of time that it takes to clear the psoriasis varies from person to person. If the plaques are very thick to begin with, it will take longer to clear them than if they are thin and not scaly. It also depends on which treatments you are using and how effectively you are applying them. Having said this, as a general rule you should reckon on 4–8 weeks of regular treatment (according to the instructions) before clearance occurs, although there will be improvement before this to encourage you. Because it takes this length of time, it is especially important for you to find a treatment that fits your lifestyle and is as easy as possible to use regularly.

Does treatment need to be ongoing?

Once your skin clears of psoriasis, you need only continue to use moisturisers (lotions are often sufficient). However, keep your eyes open for any new spots appearing as it is easier to treat these when they are new and small rather than waiting until they get bigger and thicker.

My psoriasis clears but comes back very soon – isn't there something I can do to prevent this?

Although moisturisers are all that most people need once the psoriasis clears, your problem of very early recurrence after only a short time when your skin is clear can be a problem. There are some dermatologists, especially in the USA, who use a maintenance regime. This seems to help keep the skin clear if you always get the plaques in the same places. The vitamin D creams are the most popular ones to try, but you should discuss it with your GP or consultant first. A little bit of the cream applied just at weekends to the areas of skin that have cleared often seems to be all that is needed.

What is the success rate of available treatments?

Most treatments mentioned in this chapter have a good success rate when used properly (regularly and in conjunction with moisturisers). The difficulty that many people experience lies in trying to keep up regular treatments – for example, fitting twice-daily regimes into everyday life. You may in the end decide that you are content to keep your psoriasis comfortable and under control and that complete clearance is unrealistic because the treatment regimes do not fit into your lifestyle. This point of view is fine, and you should make sure that your doctor understands that, for you, this is a reasonable success. It is very important to come to this type of understanding as your measure of success will differ from another person's and may also be different for you at different times of your life. You might be happy with some residual psoriasis that is hidden under winter clothes but not when the summer comes and you want to wear more revealing outfits. Similarly, you might want to make a big effort with the creams before an important event such as a wedding.

Does perspiration help to clear up psoriasis?

No, it doesn't. In fact, some people find that getting hot and sweating aggravates the symptoms of psoriasis by making it much more itchy.

Are there any restrictions to my treatments?

It is difficult to answer this question without knowing your exact treatments, but the following points can be made to establish some general principles. First, moisturising is a key component of treatment, and whereas it is hard to use too much moisturiser, if you use too little it will not be as effective. Further discussion about recommended amounts of moisturiser can be found later in this chapter. Most of the other treatments do have recommended amounts for usage as well as a recommended length of time over which they should be used. For example:

- **Steroids.** These should be used with caution and only over a short period of time. They are rarely used on their own for chronic plaque psoriasis because, although they initially make it better, the psoriasis can come back worse than before when the steroids are stopped (rebound effect). They are, however, useful for psoriasis that is more inflamed than usual, psoriasis in the flexures (groins, underarms and under the breasts) and on the face, although even greater care needs to be taken near the eyes. In each box of steroid, there is a guidance sheet for the correct amount to use measured in 'fingertip units' (see later in the chapter.

- **Vitamin D derivatives.** The recommended quantity for these is not more than 100 g over a period of a week in an adult. Overuse could possibly interfere with the body's absorption of calcium.

- **Coal tar/dithranol.** There is no real restriction to the amount of these that you can use, but they can make your skin sore and uncomfortable if you use more than you need. They are not recommended for the more delicate parts of your skin – i.e. your face and flexures.

Moisturisers

Why should I use moisturisers?

Although there is little scientific research into the effects of moisturisers on psoriasis, our own experience shows that:

- moisturisers make the skin *much* more comfortable – they decrease the dryness, scaling, cracking and soreness, and itching;

- moisturisers allow the other active treatments that you use (e.g. tar or vitamin D) to work more effectively.

Which moisturiser is best to use?

There are so many to choose from that it is sometimes difficult to know which to choose. There are, however, two golden rules:

- Moisturising is absolutely vital for anyone with psoriasis. Although it does not get rid of the psoriasis, it makes it less scaly and much more comfortable.

- The best moisturiser is the one that you feel happiest with and that you feel you can use easily on a regular basis. Discuss this with your GP and ask her or him to prescribe one that you like and will use. You may find that you need two or three different moisturisers for different parts of your body or different times of day, so don't be afraid to ask to try several varieties.

Below are some other things to think about when you are choosing a moisturiser.

Consistency

Lotions are water based and tend to be very runny and easy to apply (e.g. E45 lotion). They are quite cooling but not very good at moisturising, particularly dry skin. They are useful for maintaining good skin once the psoriasis has gone.

Creams are thicker and a bit greasier than lotions but are still easy to use (e.g. Diprobase). They are less runny and tend to come in pots or pump dispensers. They are usually the best option for day-to-day use.

Ointments are very greasy and thick, and are oil rather than water based (e.g. Epaderm or 50/50 white soft paraffin/liquid paraffin mix). They are the best moisturisers but are less pleasant to use because they are greasy and quite sticky. If, however, your skin is very dry, they are the best option.

Doublebase is a relatively new gel-based emollient that many people find smoothes into the skin very easily.

Frequency

You should use your moisturiser at least twice a day and more often if possible. Try to make your treatment fit in with your lifestyle as best you can. Some suggestions are to use a lighter cream moisturiser in the morning before going to work or school and then use a greasier ointment before going to bed. Try taking a small pot of cream to work with you and applying it if a patch gets particularly dry, itchy or uncomfortable. If you are applying a moisturiser all over, it is very easy to get through a 500 g pot in a week or so, so make sure that your doctor prescribes enough.

Method of application

When you apply the moisturiser, you should do this by gently stroking the cream/ointment on in a way that follows the lie of the little hairs on the skin. Try not to rub too aggressively as this will only serve to aggravate the plaques – a gentle repeated motion is best. A pump dispenser is best as it saves you having to keep putting your hand into the pot. If you have a moisturiser that does not come with a pump dispenser, scoop out what you need with a clean spoon – this stops dirt and skin scale getting into the pot.

In the bath or shower

Moisturising is not just about putting cream or ointments on: it starts in the bath or shower. As indicated in the answer to a later question, in the section 'Practical aspects', it is wise to wash with a soap substitute that does not dry your skin. If you choose to bathe, put a bath oil in the water; this helps to create a layer of oil over the skin, which prevents water being lost from the skin. Beware of the risk of slipping, though, when you get in and out of the bath or shower!

To summarise, moisturising should involve:

- using a soap substitute;
- putting an oil (e.g. Balneum, Oilatum or Diprobath) in the bath;
- using lots of cream or ointment moisturisers at least twice a day;
- choosing the moisturisers that suit you and your lifestyle best.

The final thing to remember is that moisturisers do not actually add water to the skin: they stop it being lost by evaporation from the skin. Make sure you have enough water in your body to help them do their job – don't let yourself become dehydrated.

When should I apply moisturisers?

As mentioned in the answer above, moisturisers should be applied as often as possible. There are, however, two key times when moisturisers are a must:

- straight after a bath or shower as the skin is warm and well hydrated so will absorb the moisturiser better and the extra water will be sealed into the skin;

- before putting on a treatment. It is important that the moisturiser is absorbed into the skin because, if it is sitting on the surface of the skin, it may make the active treatment less effective.

A good routine to get into is to bathe or shower using a soap substitute, apply moisturiser and allow it to sink into the skin, and then apply the active treatment. (A lotion will be absorbed almost straight away, but it can take 10–15 minutes for a cream and 45–60 minutes for an ointment to be absorbed.) You should repeat this process at either end of the day, although you clearly need to bathe or shower only once. Any other moisturiser that you can apply throughout the day is a bonus.

How much moisturiser should I apply?

You will often hear people say that you should apply moisturisers 'liberally'. The truth of the matter is that the amount you will use will depend on how big you are and how dry your skin is. It is, however, also true to say that most people do not use enough moisturiser. Some straightforward guidance is to think about applying 25 g for an all-over application each time you use moisturiser, 25 g equating to approximately five teaspoons of cream or ointment. Use one teaspoonful on each leg, half a teaspoon for each arm, one for the front of your trunk and one for the back. It is a good idea to do this at least twice a day. You will know you are using enough when your skin feels smooth and not dried out. You can easily see how you will get through 500 g in 7–10 days using this regime.

I keep hearing people talking about emollient therapy. What is this, and is there a difference between this and moisturisers?

The only difference between emollients and moisturisers is the words themselves rather than their meaning: they mean essentially the same thing. The phrase 'emollient therapy' is, however, sometimes used to refer to the whole procedure described in the answer to an earlier question – i.e. the use of soap substitutes and bath oil as well as the application of creams or ointments. In this context, 'moisturisers' usually refer to the creams and ointments themselves.

What is the difference between creams and ointments? I thought that all the things you put on your skin were creams.

Although there is a difference between creams and ointments, it can get a bit confusing because people refer to all the substances that go on the skin as creams. Strictly speaking, creams are water based, tend to be white in colour and are quickly absorbed into the skin. Although they are good moisturisers, they are not as effective as ointments, which are oil based. Ointments tend to be (although are not always) translucent, and they are very good moisturisers. So a moisturiser can be either a cream or an ointment.

But, to make life more complicated, other treatments can come in cream or ointment form. Most steroid applications, for example, come in either an ointment or a cream, as do vitamin D applications. As mentioned in an earlier answer, ointments, although they have a better moisturising effect, tend to be less pleasant to use and can take much longer to be absorbed if you need to apply an active preparation on top. The choice is personal preference, and you need to decide for yourself which preparations you like best. GPs often prescribe the ointment form of vitamin D and steroid treatments. If you find these too 'tacky' or sticky, ask your GP to prescribe you the cream form. If you are using moisturisers as well, it is less important to have the greasy form of the active treatment.

Should I be using moisturisers – my doctor has given me Dovonex?

Yes! Yes! Yes! No matter what other treatment your doctor gives you, you should always use moisturiser before applying the other treatment. The moisturiser (once it has sunk in) makes the other treatment more effective as well as easier to apply by reducing the scale and allowing a better absorption of the active creams.

Coal tar

Coal tar was the best for me. Why can't I still get it?

Many chemists have stopped making up coal tar solutions in white soft paraffin. This is because legislation has meant that they need more safety equipment to manufacture coal tar preparations, and most chemists do not have these facilities. These treatments are still available in dermatology departments but rarely in high-street chemists. Weak tar-based products such as Exorex and Cocois are still clearly available.

I used to use Alphosyl lotion with some success but now cannot find it in any pharmacy. What has happened?

Since November 2003, Alphosyl lotion has no longer been available in the UK. You may find that Exorex, which is another weak coal tar preparation, is suitable for you. Note, though, that Alphosyl 2 in 1 shampoo is still available.

I have read a lot about Exorex and understand that it is available on prescription. Is it worth trying?

Exorex is the brand name for a group of treatments for psoriasis. There is a *lotion* that is a weak tar solution (and has the characteristic tar smell), and also a *moisturiser* and a *shampoo* (which do not contain tar). Tar is a useful treatment for psoriasis and is helpful for many people. The amount of tar in Exorex is low, but the lotion is easy to put on, so some of its reported success may simply reflect the fact that people will keep using it. The cream contains an extract from the banana plant, which is what sparked a lot of media attention. It is a cream and is slightly greasy (see Appendix 3). It is really a matter of personal preference whether you like it more than any of the other emollients.

Steroids

My cousin's doctor has suggested that he might need to use steroids for his psoriasis. What do steroids actually do?

Steroids are essentially hormones, and there are many different types with quite different actions. The human body makes its own steroids in the adrenal glands, and these are vital for the body's normal function.

Different types of synthetic steroid have been developed for use in medicine. There is a group called anabolic steroids, which some athletes take (illegally!) to help build up muscle mass, and these *should not be confused* with the steroids used in psoriasis. These belong to another group called catabolic steroids or glucocorticoids (e.g. prednisolone), which are taken orally (by mouth) because of their anti-inflammatory and immunosuppressive properties – they damp down the activity of various immune cells in the body that cause inflammation. They are very useful, even life-saving, in some medical conditions such as severe asthma or rheumatoid arthritis. The downside of this group of steroids is that if they are used at a high dose *for a prolonged period*, they have many side-effects such as weight gain, bone thinning, decreased growth in children, high blood pressure and loss of muscle mass, to name but a few. Because of this, doctors try to use these steroids at the lowest possible dose for short periods. This type of oral steroid is used very occasionally in the treatment of a very severe flare-up of psoriasis. However, for the reasons already mentioned, they are normally used for only a few weeks, the starting dose being gradually decreased over this period of time. This method should prevent or minimise any serious side-effects.

Fortunately, these anti-inflammatory steroids can also be made into creams for topical application directly on to the skin (topical steroids). They act in a fashion similar to that of their oral counterparts. These creams have been developed to try to produce the same anti-inflammatory properties without all the side-effects on the rest of the body, even after long-term use. This approach has been very successful, and topical steroids are useful for psoriasis in certain circumstances such as on the scalp and in the flexures, or if the psoriasis is very inflamed.

Why is there so much conflicting information about steroids and their safety?

This is an extremely common question and worry for many people. We are not entirely sure why so much misinformation has been generated about topical steroids, but people do seem to have extremely strong views about their safety. The following points may in part explain why some of the myths have developed:

- The very earliest topical steroids developed were poorly regulated and of uncertain strength (potency). Even as late as the early 1980s, there was little recognition of the potential danger of an excessive use of the potent steroids, so there were unwanted and undesirable side-effects. These included skin thinning if used on skin other than the palms and soles for more than a few weeks. Unfortunately, when this side-effect was noticed, topical steroids got a bad name. This bad publicity has regrettably been inappropriately extended by some people to all steroids, even the very weak ones. Remember that topical steroids vary enormously in strength. (For examples of steroids, see Appendix 3.)

- Steroids taken by mouth have a number of side-effects, and many people assume that topical steroids do as well. This is not true. Topical steroids were developed specifically to prevent the problems of oral steroids.

- There are different types of steroid, which act differently and have different side-effects. It is easy to assume that all steroids are the same and thus misunderstand the side-effect risks. For example, anabolic steroids can cause an increase in muscle size and liver damage but this *does not* occur with the topical steroids used in psoriasis. Anabolic steroids are not available as creams, so there is no chance of being given the wrong type.

- Many people have become disillusioned with conventional medicine. There has been a social trend to assume that Western medicines are dangerous and that herbal remedies or natural products are safe and preferable. The word 'steroid' has become almost synonymous with all that is bad about conventional medical treatments.

- Steroids do not cure psoriasis, so it often recurs after using them and can 'rebound' (come back) and become worse. You may have expected a cure – partly because the media love reporting on 'miracle cures' – and might be reluctant to use them again.

We would not claim that any conventional therapy is 100% safe, but then neither are less conventional treatments. Risks have to be assessed for any form of therapy. Provided that topical steroids are used appropriately, they are an extremely valuable, safe and effective part of psoriasis therapy. It is interesting that in the USA, where patients are much more likely to sue over adverse effects, dermatologists use more steroid therapy for psoriasis than we do in the UK.

What does 'use sparingly' on my box of steroid ointment mean?

Each box should come with a chart giving details of the correct amount to use, in 'fingertip units'. This indicates the safe and correct amount of steroid to apply by using the length of the tip of your finger (the section after the last joint) to measure out the steroid. If you are using steroid creams or ointments in a very small area – for example, just under your arms – apply a thin layer and rub it in well. 'Sparingly' is not really a very useful term: doctors should try to be more precise and give you more useful directions. As a general rule, 'sparingly' could be taken to mean the least amount that will do the job.

Vitamin D

My husband's doctor has suggested trying vitamin D treatment. What does this do?

This refers to topical applications that contain vitamin D derivatives and have been very helpful in the treatment of milder forms of psoriasis. Vitamin D is essential for the healthy growth of the skin. The topical vitamin D applications (e.g. Dovonex) are less messy than dithranol and tar, and many people find them very effective! They are available as creams, ointments and scalp applications.

For the treatment to be effective, it is important to apply a 'thick smear' and then gently rub it in. A 'thick smear' means covering the area with cream or ointment so that you can see it on your skin before rubbing it in. Vitamin D creams *do not* need to be used 'sparingly', as do steroid creams and ointments, as long as you do not use more than 100 g a week.

Should I take a course of vitamin D?

No. Vitamins should be present in a normal healthy diet, and taking supplements will have little or no effect on the skin.

I have noticed that, since I started using my new vitamin D cream, my eyes have become very sore. Is there any link?

This is probably caused by you rubbing your eyes (or even just touching them) after you have applied the vitamin D cream to your body. It is very important that, after applying any of the active treatments, you wash your hands thoroughly to make sure that they are clear of any trace of the treatment. As you have discovered, even the smallest amount can cause irritation when it comes into contact with your face or eyes. This advice is especially important if you also use steroids as they are unlikely to cause irritation but might cause damage if repeatedly rubbed into or around the eyes, even accidentally.

What is Dovobet?

Dovobet is the trade name for a topical treatment that combines a potent steroid with calcipotriol (Dovonex). It is generally used for plaque psoriasis and is initially prescribed for 4 weeks. It appears to work more quickly than Dovonex, but, owing to the fact that it contains potent steroid, it should not be used for prolonged periods of time. The maximum dose is 100 g per week.

Different treatments for different areas

I have areas of psoriasis on my knees, and the doctor has recommended that I use short-contact Dithrocream. I don't really understand what I have to do.

Dithrocream is a type of dithranol that is very helpful in treating well-defined and easily accessible areas of psoriasis, such as those on the elbows and knees. The 'short-contact' approach has been designed for use at home as it is less messy than the paste forms of dithranol used in hospital. It involves applying gradually increasing strengths of Dithrocream to the plaques of psoriasis and leaving the cream in place before washing it off (best done in the shower or bath). Apply enough to cover the plaque completely, and rub the cream in until it is completely absorbed. The first strength is usually 0.1%, followed by 0.25%, and going up to 2%. One reason for gradually increasing the strength is to minimise the likelihood of your skin becoming sore. The Dithrocream must be applied carefully to the plaques, not the good skin, making sure that it does not smudge. It should then be washed off after half an hour and moisturisers reapplied. This only needs to be done once a day. Always remember to wash your hands thoroughly after applying treatment. You may wish to wear plastic gloves to avoid staining your fingertips.

Some people find that the very weak strengths have little or no effect. If this is the case for you, you should move quickly to the next strength up, spending no more than 3 or 4 days at the lower strengths. If you find your skin getting sore, you could either return to a lower strength or discontinue the treatment – it really depends on how sore it is, and this is clearly an individual judgement. Uniquely, all five strengths of Dithrocream can be prescribed on one prescription and you will only have to pay one prescription charge, so ask your GP to do this. There is another form of dithranol for short-contact treatment – this is called Micanol, but it only comes in two strengths. It may be less likely to stain baths and showers when washing it off.

I have psoriasis in the genital area. Can I use the same ointment as I have for my elbows and knees?

In general, your doctor will prescribe you different creams for your knees/elbows and for your genital area. The skin in the genital area is thinner and therefore more sensitive than that on your elbows/knees so is more likely to be irritated. Using the same treatment there may actually cause damage and soreness. There is also the fact that the genital area tends to be warm and moist, which means that the treatment is absorbed more readily and therefore does not need to be as strong to be effective. Mild-to-moderate-potency steroids are often used in the genital and other flexural areas (e.g. the armpits) and, because infections with yeasts and bacteria are common in these places, are often combined with antifungal and antibacterial agents.

Which is the best treatment to put on my scalp?

The treatment that you use on your scalp will depend very much on the extent to which it is affected and what you want to achieve:

- **Coconut oil.** This is good if your scalp is dry but not necessarily covered with active psoriasis. The coconut oil is solid at room temperature but melts on contact with the skin and is therefore quite greasy; it has a very light but not unpleasant smell. Use as much as you need to make your scalp feel comfortable. Olive oil or some of the bath oil you might have been prescribed can also be used. This can be applied overnight under a shower cap and can be very effective at removing scale, allowing some of the more active treatments to work.

- **Coal tar solution (Cocois).** If the psoriasis on your scalp is thick and active, this is the best treatment to use as it moistens the plaques and encourages them to lift off. Because it has tar in it, it does tend to be a bit messy and has a distinctive smell. The amount you need to use will depend on how thick your psoriasis is, but apply enough to turn the scale from white to the colour of the ointment. As with the oils, you might want to wear a shower cap to prevent staining the pillows as it is a good treatment to leave on overnight.

- **Steroid (e.g. Betnovate) scalp application.** This is useful for short-term treatment if the scalp is inflamed but the plaques are not particularly thick. It is relatively clean and odour free. Beware, though: the scalp application is an alcohol based solution and can sting when applied. There is a mousse-style preparation available if the stinging is a problem for you.

- **Vitamin D scalp application.** This is useful when the plaques are thin but active. It is clean and odour free. One or two drops are enough to cover an area of your head about the size of a postage stamp.

It is very difficult to apply my scalp treatment. Have you any advice?

With scalp treatment, the method of application is almost as important as which treatment you use. Applying the treatment involves parting the hair in sections and rubbing the treatment along the exposed area. It is best to do this in a sequential fashion, starting at the front of the scalp and working your way round. If the scale/plaques are very thick, they can be gently lifted up using a comb once they have been moisturised with the treatment (especially with Cocois).

It is easier to get someone else to do this for you as it is difficult to see the top of your own head to (a) rub the treatment in where it is needed and (b) lift the scale where appropriate. When doing this, some hair may come out, but this will grow back, so don't be too perturbed! The best time to do a scalp treatment is before going to bed as the treatment (especially Cocois and coconut oil) will make your hair look greasy and can smell. Try wearing a cotton 'night cap', a shower cap or something similar, and cover your pillows with old pillowcases to protect them. (You can buy pillowcase protectors, which give useful extra protection to your pillows, from bed linen shops or departments.) Wash your hair the next morning with an anti-psoriasis (i.e. tar-based) shampoo. An advantage of the coconut-based treatments is that they are wonderful conditioners for your hair!

Once you have removed the scale, you can move on to a creamier treatment like vitamin D, which can be applied in the morning. Some people find that a combination approach works best, applying the greasy descaler at night and the creamier vitamin D in the morning after washing their hair.

What can I do treatment-wise to help get rid of psoriasis on my face?

First, apply lots of moisturiser because this will help keep the scaling under control as well as making your face more comfortable. A weak topical steroid will often help. Psoriasis on the hairline will respond to a weak coal tar preparation such as

Exorex, but it is best not to use this type on your face as it can cause discomfort. Tacalcitol (Curatoderm) and calcitriol (Silkis) are two of the vitamin D creams that are thought to be suitable for use on the face without too much irritation. Whichever treatment you use on your face, be very careful not to get it in your eyes.

If the psoriasis on your face does not respond to either of these treatments, it is worth consulting your doctor again in case there is a fungal or yeast component to the psoriasis (known as sebor-rhoeic psoriasis). If this is the case, you will need an antifungal cream or perhaps an antifungal and steroid cream combined.

I am so embarrassed about the psoriasis on my face. It's making me really depressed and I don't want to go out.

If you have tried the above treatments and they are not working, there are two further things that you might like to discuss with your doctor. The first is to consider using specialist camouflage make-up, which the Red Cross can teach you how to use. This service is provided free of charge, and your GP can refer you, although you will have to pay a prescription charge for the make-up. These techniques are very successful, and you may find that covering up your psoriasis in this way gives you the confidence to get out and about again. The next thing to consider is talking to your GP about going on to second-line treatments (described in Chapter 5). Although the potential side-effects are greater than for first-line treatments, you need to think about all the possible options if your psoriasis is affecting your mental health and happiness.

Practical aspects

I have been given Dithrocream, which is making a mess of the bathroom.

It is true that Dithrocream can make a mess of your bathroom, with purple stains. To stop this happening, you need to be very careful not to get the Dithrocream anywhere but on your body. To help to minimise the staining on your bath or shower when you wash the

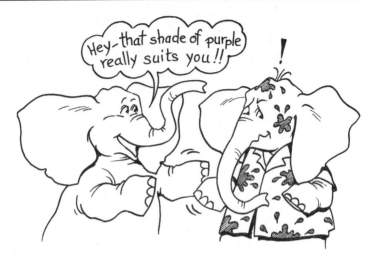

Dithrocream off, you can use cotton wool soaked in baby oil to wipe the cream off before getting into the bath or shower. Just take care not to wipe the Dithrocream on to unaffected skin. It is also worth washing round the bath or shower immediately after you have finished. If the difficulties you are having with the Dithrocream mean that you are not using the treatment, you need to see your doctor to discuss the possibility of being prescribed another one that you do feel able to use. The alternative dithranol preparation called Micanol is supposed not to have the same potential for staining the bath if washed off in lukewarm water.

The scalp lotion I am using is making my forehead so sore. Can I use something else?

You can, of course, ask your doctor to prescribe something else for your scalp. It is, however, worth considering two possible reasons why your forehead is so sore. First, are you applying your treatment properly? If you get someone else to do it for you, you may find that they do not get so much on your forehead so it stops being sore. Second, try to establish for sure that it is the treatment that is making it so sore and not the psoriasis itself. If it is actually the psoriasis that is making your forehead sore, you will need to get a specific treatment for this. A mild steroid or tar application may be appropriate. The other thing to try is a layer of moisturiser on your forehead as a kind of barrier cream before you apply the scalp lotion.

Can overuse of a special shampoo (e.g. Polytar) be harmful?

There is no evidence to show that it is. However, it is not sensible to overuse any treatment, so we strongly suggest that you use the shampoo only as often as it recommends on the bottle.

I don't think my creams work as well as they used to. Am I getting resistant to them?

There can be reasons why creams do not seem to be as effective as they used to be. One is that they might be out of date or have 'gone off'. Creams do not last for ever, especially once they have been opened, so check with your pharmacist to see whether you should request a new one. Another reason might be that a new outbreak of psoriasis might not respond to the same cream that helped the previous one. This can be very frustrating, especially if you try to treat it as soon as it starts. On the other hand, something that did not work well last time might be just right this time.

Some people report that using the same prescribed treatment for a long period of time makes it less effective. There is no scientific evidence for this except in the case of topical steroids, where long-term use can lead to a wearing off of the benefit and the need for a stronger preparation to achieve the same effect. We call this problem 'tachyphylaxis'. This is another reason why we recommend steroids only for short-term use.

The skin around the bits where I have psoriasis burns if I get the cream on them. What can I do to stop it?

The first and most obvious thing to say is that you should be very careful when you apply the cream to ensure that you get it *only* on the plaques. There are, however, two other strategies that might also help.

The first strategy is to apply a thicker layer of moisturiser around the plaques to protect the skin. This is particularly effective if you are using a thick, greasy moisturiser. In order to do this successfully, apply the moisturiser as you would do normally, allow it to sink in, then apply the prescribed topical treatment to the plaques, and then carefully apply another, thicker layer of moisturiser around each plaque. This is quite time-consuming but will be helpful.

Second, try to minimise the amount of smudging that occurs from the plaque on to the skin that has no psoriasis on it. If you are using a vitamin D cream or a weak tar-based preparation, you can do this by ensuring that you rub the treatment in well and do not put your clothes on until it has been completely absorbed. If you are using short-contact Dithrocream, it is best not to put any clothes on while the Dithrocream is on; if you do put something on, make sure it is very loose and not going to smudge the cream. The other thing to remember about smudging is that if you apply a treatment to your groin, under your arms or under your breasts, it may go on to the adjoining unaffected area. The best thing to do in this instance is to make sure that you use a treatment that will not irritate your skin (e.g. a mild topical steroid) and cover the unaffected skin with moisturiser.

Should I use soap on the areas of psoriasis?

Soap tends to have a drying effect on the skin. The soaps that are advertised as having moisturisers in them are better than others but can still have a drying effect. With this in mind, it is better to find an alternative to soap (i.e. a soap substitute). The one that is often recommended is aqueous cream, which is available from the pharmacist or on prescription, but there are others that you can buy over the counter (e.g. E45 wash). Rather than removing the protective layer of natural oils on your skin as soap does, soap substitutes serve to protect and supplement this. Another, greasier, option is emulsifying ointment. The soap substitute can then be used like a soap, applying it to the body using a wash-cloth or just your hands and then rinsing it off.

To avoid getting water and skin scales into your pot of cream or ointment, it is a good idea to scoop out, with a clean spoon, all that you are going to need for your bath or shower before you start washing. An even better idea is to get a cream in a pump dispenser, which will allow you to use as much as you need without getting water or skin scales into the pot. If you use emulsifying ointment to wash with, it is a good idea to dissolve the ointment in really hot water first before 'whisking' it into your bath or washing water – it makes a good lather and leaves your skin feeling well moisturised.

If you feel the soap substitute is not cleansing you adequately in the groin area or under your arms, use small amounts of soap there. It is worth noting that using soap substitutes to wash with should not be seen as a substitute for using a moisturiser once you have had your bath or shower and dried your skin.

Do I have to bandage up the affected skin?

No, you don't have to. Nevertheless, depending on which treatment you are using, covering the skin with tubular bandages (e.g. Tubifast) may be helpful. Particularly if you are using tar-based treatments, these types of bandage keep the treatment on your skin, where it should be, and can stop it from getting on to your clothes. Tubular bandages are stretchy cotton bandages that form a sleeve, unlike normal bandages, which need to be wrapped round. They come in different sizes to fit arms, legs and trunk, and are now available on prescription.

I am breast-feeding my baby daughter and have psoriasis on my breast. Should I stop using the cream the doctor gave me?

You should make sure, first of all, that you have told your doctor that you are breast-feeding; the doctor will then make sure that anything prescribed is safe for both you and your baby. You should make sure that, whenever you breast-feed, your nipples in particular are clear of any active treatments as these could have a damaging effect on your baby if any got into her mouth. It is important, however, that you keep the skin on your breasts as supple as possible to prevent cracks forming – especially around the nipple – so you must continue to use your treatment.

Do be aware that, although it is only your nipples that the baby is likely to suck, she will touch the rest of the skin on your breasts. She might therefore come into contact with the topical treatment you have put on – which can be damaging to delicate baby skin. It may be simplest while breast-feeding to stick to moisturisers alone, but do discuss this with your doctor.

Treatments for psoriatic arthropathy

What are the usual treatments for psoriatic arthropathy?

In general, the treatments are the same as for other sorts of arthritis and can be divided into first-line and second-line, as with treatment of the skin. The first-line treatments can be started by your GP without the need for specialist advice. In the early stages, it does not matter very much if the diagnosis has not been confirmed because the treatment will be the same for any person with joint pains.

- **Physiotherapy** is often forgotten or used only at later stages of the disease, but it can be very useful both to treat pain and stiffness and to educate you about exercises, correct lifting techniques and other simple things that can help to prevent further problems. It is a shame that there are often long waiting times to see NHS physiotherapists when all that might be needed is this simple advice. The Psoriatic Arthropathy Alliance (PAA) is a useful patient support group to contact for advice.

- **Non-steroidal anti-inflammatory drugs** (NSAIDs) are a class of drug that have been derived from aspirin, and they have a wide range of uses. In arthritis, NSAIDs are used early to relieve pain by working against the inflammation, so they also relieve swelling and stiffness. There are many different types and strengths, starting with ibuprofen – which is probably the best known as it was the first one to be available without a prescription, as Nurofen. They have some side-effects, the most important of which is irritation of the stomach; this sometimes leads to ulceration, so you should not buy them to use long term without discussing it with your GP. They should also be used with great care if you have a history of asthma as they could make this worse. (NSAIDs are also available as creams and gels to rub directly into the skin over a joint, but this is an expensive way of using the drug with little definite evidence that it works.)

- **Steroid injections.** Although steroid tablets should be seen as a second-line treatment, injections directly into a joint can be used earlier if only one large joint, such as a knee, is affected. Pain relief and a return of mobility can be very rapid, and there is only a risk of the general side-effects of steroids if the injections are given too often. This should not happen because other types of treatment would then be indicated. Many GPs are very good at giving injections and will happily do it, but others might refer you to a specialist if they do not feel confident and have not had much practice with this type of treatment. Don't put pressure on your GP to try an injection if he or she does not want to do it – it is not a 'core skill' that all GPs are expected to have.

If these simple treatments fail to help your symptoms, there are other approaches to treating arthritis with drugs that act against it to prevent inflammation and damage to the joints. These are called 'disease-modifying antirheumatic drugs – known more simply as DMARDs – and are covered in the next chapter.

5
Second-line treatment

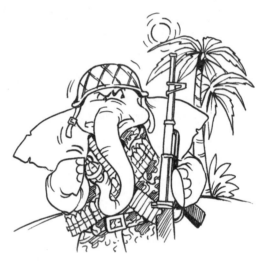

Introduction

The term 'second-line' refers to a treatment that would not be used in the first attempt to treat a patient unless the psoriasis were very severe right from the start. This is usually because the second-line treatment involves attending hospital, as either an out-patient or an in-patient, takes up more of the person's time and may have more side-effects. There are some very effective treatments that have to be 'held in reserve' in case the disease becomes more widespread or aggressive as only a limited amount can be used because of potential side-effects. Thus, if one of these were used for psoriasis that was not severe, it might not be an option when it was really needed. Ultraviolet treatment is the best example of this because the total dose given over a lifetime needs to be limited to minimise the risk of skin cancer.

Although many second-line treatments can produce side-effects serious enough to mean that the treatment has to be stopped, all these effects are very well understood. They can be minimised by careful monitoring using blood and other tests so that treatment is stopped safely before any permanent damage is done. It can, therefore, be much safer to take a well-researched powerful drug for which the dangers are known and understood than some complementary therapies involving herbs for which the dangers may be just as great but are not recognised or looked for.

In hospital

I have to go into hospital soon. What sort of treatment may I expect?

This depends to a certain extent on your consultant and the reasons for your admission to hospital. It is probably reasonable for us to assume that your psoriasis is widespread and causing you a lot of problems, otherwise you would not be admitted. In this case, it is likely that you will be having treatments and investigations. One hospital treatment, called Ingram's method, consists of dithranol paste and ultraviolet (UV) light. Specialist dermatology (skin) nurses will apply the paste to your psoriasis and bandage you up to keep the paste in contact with your skin for several hours. When it is removed, you will have UV treatment. This is done once a day and can improve the psoriasis very quickly.

It can be very good for you to have a rest from the daily grind of putting your own treatments on, and some hospitals now have special day therapy units where this can be done for you without the need to be admitted. It is, however, a great problem for some dermatology departments to hang on to their specialist in-patient facilities as the managers need to save money and view skin disease as an out-patient problem. Being admitted to a general medical ward with all sorts of different patients and nurses who lack the special training to deal with your problems can be very disheartening and may mean that you do not get the care you need. If this applies to your hospital, ask whether day care is an alternative and write to your MP! Self-help groups are usually experienced in putting pressure on hospitals and MPs, and should be able to help you phrase a suitable letter.

I recently went into hospital and had the same creams applied to my skin that had failed at home. They worked well – why is this?

If you are admitted to a specialist ward where the staff are properly trained in looking after skin problems, it can be a very restful place. Add to this the chance to relax and avoid any household chores and it is not surprising that treatments work better! You mentioned that creams were applied to your skin for you – this also makes a difference, as you do not have to worry about finding the time or making sure that the creams do not make marks or stains around the house. Many people also enjoy the touching involved as this can be sadly lacking when you have a skin disease. Some people describe hospital as a place of sanctuary – somewhere safe to escape to – which seems to describe an ideal to be aimed for by all hospitals.

It is also worth considering whether you had been applying the right amount of treatment while you were at home. Commonly, people do not apply the right amount of creams and ointments, and this is why they do not work. In hospital, the nurses will have been trained to use the correct amount, which might help to explain why they were more effective during your stay on the ward.

I hate going into hospital to get my psoriasis under control. Is there no alternative?

It depends what you mean by 'going into' hospital. If you mean being admitted and staying over one or more nights, this is becoming much more unusual as many hospital departments now have day-care centres where you go to have treatments applied by the nurses but go home each night. This may involve wearing bandages to cover the creams, but it could be a suitable option if you do not want to stay overnight. If you really hate the idea of even going to a day centre, you will have to discuss this with your consultant to see whether any of the other treatments mentioned in this chapter would be suitable for you. The stress you might feel while in hospital might work against the benefits of the treatment.

Ultraviolet light treatment

Why is natural sunlight such a good healer?

Natural sunlight is a good healer for many people with psoriasis, but there are some who do not respond and some who are made worse. Sunlight consists of several different types of light across a spectrum ranging from infrared through visible light to UV. It is the UV part that can help in treating psoriasis.

The skin cells contain specialised molecules (called chromophores) that are capable of absorbing the energy from UV light and then releasing it to power chemical reactions that affect the function of the cells. In psoriasis, this can result in the cells not multiplying as rapidly and behaving more like normal skin.

Should I buy a sunbed?

'No' is the quick answer to this question! Although UV light can help some people with psoriasis, and even if you have noticed your skin getting better on holiday, there are dangers in using sunbeds. UV light can lead to the development of skin cancers, and dermatologists (skin specialists) would advise against anyone using a sunbed. When you have psoriasis, controlled UV treatment can be very effective in clearing your skin, but if you use a sunbed it will be impossible for the hospital to calculate a safe dosage of UV for your skin and for you to be sure that you are getting the right type of UV light. Most sunbeds emit predominantly UVA, which is not effective on its own for psoriasis.

What is PUVA?

PUVA is a light treatment using a **p**soralen and **UVA**. Natural sunlight contains different types of UV light labelled 'A' and 'B'

(UVA and UVB). UVA on its own is not active in skin disease, but if given with a 'psoralen' (which makes the skin more sensitive to light – photosensitive) it can be very effective. The psoralen, which is derived from plants, is sometimes taken by mouth but can be applied via a bath containing the chemical; alternatively, small areas can be treated using a topical paint. Not all people with psoriasis will benefit from PUVA. The bath application is becoming more popular as it causes fewer problems related to the psoralen getting into the body and seems to need a shorter exposure time for each treatment session.

The use of UV light in the UK is governed by guidelines from the British Photodermatology Group, which looks at what groups of people should be treated and decides on safe dosages. It has identified three main groups of people who should be considered for PUVA treatment:

- people with severe psoriasis that is not responding to topical treatments;

- people whose psoriasis returns within 3–6 months of successful treatment as an in-patient or at a day centre;

- people who do not want topical treatment and for whom UVB has failed to produce enough of a clearing response.

Why do I need to wear sunglasses on the days I have PUVA?

When the psoralen is taken by mouth, it is absorbed through the gut and affects more than just the skin. The eyes are also made more sensitive to light, which can cause cataracts to develop. To protect your eyes, you must wear glasses that filter out the UV rays as soon as you take the tablet. These need to be worn for the rest of the day. If you feel uncomfortable wearing sunglasses all day, you can get spectacles with clear glass that filters out UV light, but make absolutely certain they are the right type. You should be able to get your glasses tested, to make sure that they are filtering out the UV rays, in the dermatology department where you are having the UVA therapy.

More and more people are having the psoralen applied directly to the skin by lying in a solution of it in a bath before the UVA treatment. Even then, enough of the drug may be absorbed to make the eyes sensitive and at risk, so sunglasses are still needed.

I have had PUVA treatment but it seems that my psoriasis has got worse. Why is this?

There might be a couple of ways to explain this. Most patients with psoriasis can be helped by UV treatment, but some are not and some do get worse. This is usually obvious from the pattern of your psoriasis: if you get worse in summer and better in winter, extra UV light is not for you. The other explanation relates to the severity of your psoriasis. If it is bad and going through a natural cycle of getting worse, any treatment might seem to fail. If you mean that your psoriasis improved or cleared with PUVA and then recurred in a more severe form later on, there is unlikely to be a link with the treatment.

Why do doctors offer treatments like PUVA with a slight risk involved when the end result isn't very good?

We would hope that the days in which doctors were accused of playing 'god' are gone. Nowadays, the relationship between you and your doctor should be much more of a partnership as you have a right to know about all the available treatments and the risks involved, so that you can play your part in deciding which one is best for you at any given time. We used to use the term 'compliance' to mean the way in which a patient stuck to the instructions for using a treatment, but now we use 'concordance' to indicate an agreement between the patient and the doctor about how to treat and which treatment to use. You should be able to discuss with your doctor the benefits and possible risks associated with any treatment offered to you. Few options are risk-free, and the final decision about whether to go ahead should be yours.

PUVA and its risks are very well understood, and for most people it can work well, clearing the skin and delaying the return of the psoriasis. All patients having PUVA are carefully counselled about the risks, and most of them agree that they are acceptable. Most of the risk comes from the UV light, but in some circumstances the psoralen can cause problems. If there is a chance of damage to the liver from heavy drinking or because of a history of jaundice, the psoralen can cause extra damage. In such instances, blood tests are needed to make sure that the liver is working normally before using the treatment.

Psoriasis is a tricky condition to treat because it can vary in its response to treatment – not just between people but also between different attacks in the same person. You might not respond well to PUVA on one occasion, but it could work better in the future. Because of this variation, we need as many different ways of treating patients as possible.

It is also very useful to be able to use treatments like PUVA to give people a break from the daily grind of applying creams. We once heard a consultant describe his patients as being 'war weary' from the constant battle with their psoriasis. In studies of people's attitudes to psoriasis and the risk of treatment, many patients preferred to take a tablet with some side-effects if it worked and cleared their psoriasis. The general comment was that to live to 65 with no psoriasis would be a lot better than to live to 75 with psoriasis!

I have been offered narrow-band UVB treatment. What does this mean?

UVB contains quite a wide range of wavelengths (290–320 nanometres (nm)), and although it can be useful in guttate psoriasis (described Chapter 1), it has never been as useful as PUVA for other types. In the past few years, a more defined form of UVB (311 nm) has been developed – hence the name 'narrow-band'. This seems to be almost as effective as PUVA without all the drawbacks of taking the psoralen. It is, therefore, much easier to use, and although PUVA may have a slightly higher rate of success, if your skin clears with narrow-band UVB it will stay clear (in remission) as long as it would have done with PUVA. You would have the treatment in the same way as PUVA, by standing in a special cabinet containing UVB tubes – like fluorescent light tubes but made to emit only the

UVB. Each treatment course would involve a session every 2 or 3 days for 5–8 weeks.

Is narrow-band UVB treatment safer than PUVA?

Yes it is. Because you are not using a psoralen, you will not have any of the possible side-effects of that, including the risk of developing cataracts if you did not wear the special glasses on treatment days. It can, therefore, be used in children and in women who are pregnant. It is still thought to increase the risk of skin cancer but not the dangerous melanoma type (PUVA does increase the risk of melanoma and other types of skin cancer). Because of this, you could have more UVB sessions than PUVA sessions – 450 compared with between 150 and 200. Some people with very difficult psoriasis may need more than the maximum number of sessions of PUVA, and they are recommended to visit the dermatologist once every year just to have their skin checked for signs of cancer.

How do the doctors know how much UV light to give me?

This is a good question as we all vary in our reaction to UV light – as you can see on any beach in the summer! The dose of UV light used in narrow-band UVB and PUVA is worked out from the lowest amount that will turn your type of skin red (redness being called 'erythema'). This is known as the 'minimum erythema dose' (MED) in UVB and 'minimum phototoxic dose' (MPD) for PUVA as the added effect of the psoralen has to be accounted for. The redness lasts for 48–72 hours, so treatment is usually given two or three times a week to allow the skin to recover between doses. The starting dose is set at 70% of the MED or MPD and is increased depending on the reaction to each treatment. If your skin does not show any redness, the next treatment will be 40% more than the previous one, but a little redness will reduce this increase to 20%. Once you start reacting to the treatment it will be held at the same dose, but as you progress through a course the dose is slowly increased to compensate for the tanning effect, which starts to block some of the UV light.

Is there any need to use my creams when having UV treatment?

It is well worth using a moisturiser regularly as the treatment may tend to make your skin dry, but most people like to have a rest from applying the active creams. If you are having UVB and it is not working as well as it might, the doctor might suggest using one of the active creams in between treatment sessions. UVB has been shown to work well in combination with coal tar, dithranol, vitamin D derivatives and retinoid cream. There is also some evidence that applying a moisturiser before your UVB session helps the treatment to work.

Methotrexate

My wife's doctor has prescribed methotrexate. Is it a steroid?

No, methotrexate (MTX) is a drug that acts to stop rapid or excessive cell growth – a 'cytotoxic' agent. It stops the rapid turnover of skin cells that cause the typical plaques of psoriasis. Unfortunately, it does not just act on the skin, so care has to be taken to avoid damage to other organs, especially the liver. It can also affect the bone marrow, where most of the blood cells are made, so regular tests are necessary to pick this up before it becomes a real problem.

I have heard that methotrexate is a drug originally developed for the treatment of cancer. If so, is there any connection between the two conditions, and is the effect of methotrexate the same in both conditions?

There is no connection between the two conditions in that neither is more common if you suffer from the other. Both psoriasis and cancer, however, involve cells growing and multiplying more rapidly than they should, so the cytotoxic action of methotrexate has the same effect on those cells. It can be used because cells that are growing normally are not as sensitive to the drug as are abnormal ones.

I take methotrexate and understand it can affect the liver. Are there any long-term problems from taking this drug?

Damage to the liver can occur with the long-term use of methotrexate, but it can also affect the bone marrow and interfere with the production of blood cells. The drug tends to be used in low doses in psoriasis so does not cause many other problems. In the higher doses used in some cancer treatments (chemotherapy), it can have toxic effects on the lungs and gut.

Why do I have to have a liver biopsy – wouldn't a blood test be enough?

Methotrexate can damage the liver, and as the side-effects are well known, doctors like to be able to avoid or prevent them. If you waited for signs of liver damage to show up in the blood, you might have developed long-term problems. The liver biopsy, which involves using a wide needle to take a small sample of the liver tissue, can show some very early and subtle changes before they do you any harm. There are, of course, some risks of having a liver biopsy, and you usually need to spend a day in hospital in case of internal bleeding; this added risk is taken into consideration when weighing up the pros and cons of using the treatment. Liver biopsies are not done very often, maybe only every couple of years depending on the dose you need.

Recent research has suggested that a blood test for a substance called 'pro-collagen 3' may be able to indicate the presence of any liver damage accurately enough to prevent the need for a liver biopsy. The test should soon become generally available, but careful monitoring will be needed to make sure that it is safe to rely on.

Does methotrexate interfere with other drugs?

There are some problems with methotrexate and other drugs that you may be prescribed or buy over the counter that tend to make the methotrexate more toxic. The common drugs are trimethoprim (an antibiotic often used for urinary infections), phenytoin (a drug for epilepsy), aspirin and other anti-inflammatory drugs such as ibuprofen, some 'water' tablets (diuretics) used to treat high blood pressure and heart failure, and the retinoid drugs such as Neotigason (mentioned below).

I am doing very well on methotrexate as it keeps my skin almost clear. Why do I have to keep going to the hospital for a prescription?

Although methotrexate can be prescribed by GPs, it is a drug that they do not have to use very often and one that has potentially very serious side-effects. This means that GPs may not be happy to take the responsibility for prescribing it in case errors are made or they do not spot any potential problems soon enough. In the NHS, it is the doctor who prescribes a medicine who is responsible for any problems, even if it is prescribed after advice from the hospital. We know of several cases where the dose has been changed to daily rather than weekly, so the patients received seven times the desired dose – or could have if they themselves or alert pharmacists had not noticed the mistake.

Under changes to GPs' contracts in 2004, it could be much safer for GPs to take on the prescribing of methotrexate and other second-line drugs normally prescribed in hospital. As long as they can demonstrate a good understanding of the drugs, side-effects and monitoring requirements, they will be able to attract an extra payment to run a clinic to look after patients on these drugs. The extra money will cover the cost of extra nursing time and the blood tests. This is called 'near patient testing' as the prescription and blood tests will be done locally rather than needing a trip to hospital.

Does having taken methotrexate in the past affect my chances of getting pregnant?

This depends on how long ago you stopped taking the drug. Methotrexate does affect the rate of production of eggs in women and of sperm in men, as well as causing abnormalities in the growing baby in the womb and increasing the risk of miscarriage if you are still taking it when you get pregnant. As long as you have waited for at least one full menstrual cycle after stopping methotrexate, you will have the same chances of a successful pregnancy as you had before starting it. Although men can father normal children while they are taking methotrexate, it is usually a good idea not to try until at least 3 months after stopping.

I feel very sick when I take methotrexate. Is there anything that can stop this?

This is the most common side-effect as up to 25% of people taking methotrexate may have the same problem as you. You have probably found that it comes on about 12 hours after taking the tablet and can last up to 3 days, so even though it is described as 'mild' in most cases, it can be a great nuisance. There are no sure-fire ways to stop the sick feeling (nausea), but the vitamin folic acid, taken every day, helps most people. Other suggestions that have helped some people include increasing the amount of water you drink in the 24 hours before taking the tablets, taking them with your evening meal and even eating a banana with the dose!

Can I still use my creams when I start methotrexate?

Yes. There are no problems with any of the topical treatments used in psoriasis. Drugs taken by mouth that might affect the immune system and UV light treatments should, however, be avoided.

Vitamin A

I've read that vitamin A treatment is good. What is it all about?

Otherwise known as retinoids, vitamin A-derived treatments can be very helpful with moderate-to-severe psoriasis. Neotigason (acitretin) is the (oral) drug name you are most likely to encounter.

There are a number of side (unwanted) effects with this class of drug, as well as some circumstances when it should not be used. Because it is teratogenic (it damages the unborn child), it should be given only in exceptional circumstances to women of child-bearing age. It can also cause nausea, dryness of the mucous membranes (mainly the eyes and lips) and temporary hair loss. A cream derived from vitamin A is also available (Zorac [tazarotene]) and is a useful addition to the treatments on offer, although it can also cause dryness and irritation of the skin.

Should I take a course of vitamin A?

No. Vitamins should be present in a normal healthy diet, and taking supplements will have little or no effect on the skin, whatever some adverts may claim. Vitamin A in particular is harmful if taken to excess, especially if you are pregnant. It can cause liver damage.

I have been taking Neotigason tablets for 2 years and now I am thinking of trying for a baby. How long will I have to wait before the effects have worn off?

Neotigason is a retinoid drug derived from vitamin A and is very useful in some forms of psoriasis. Unfortunately, it can lead to severe deformities in a developing baby, so you must not take it when pregnant. The drug persists in the body in very small amounts for a long time, and as this would be enough to cause the damage, you should wait for 2 years after stopping treatment before trying for a baby.

We hope that this was properly explained to you before you started the treatment. It is good practice for doctors to ask women to sign a consent form before starting the drug, to show that they have been given, and have understood, a full explanation of the effects and the absolute need for contraceptive precautions if they are of child-bearing age. Barrier methods of contraception, such as condoms, are not thought to be safe enough, so most women are expected to take the contraceptive pill.

My husband is taking Neotigason. Is it safe for us to try for a baby?

Although Neotigason can harm developing babies, it does not affect the production of sperm and does not cause changes to the genetic material. So it is safe for you to try for a baby.

My consultant has offered me PUVA as well as Neotigason as the latter hasn't worked on its own. Isn't this risky?

Treatment using a retinoid (Neotigason) and **PUVA** is called **RePUVA.** The combination works quite well but is usually reserved for difficult cases – such as when there is little improvement after 50 PUVA treatments, when the psoriasis returns within 6 months of successful PUVA treatment or when there is severe psoriasis of the palms and soles. The advantages of using this combination are that the retinoid can decrease the total amount of UV exposure needed and that it also acts to prevent some of the skin changes that might lead to cancer.

Ciclosporin

Why have I been offered treatment with ciclosporin? I have a friend who takes this because he has had a kidney transplant.

The use of ciclosporin reflects the importance of your immune system in the psoriatic process. It is a drug that is used to alter the body's immune response and hence helps to prevent the rejection of transplants. A transplant patient with psoriasis noticed that the psoriasis improved dramatically with ciclosporin, and it was tried with success in non-transplant patients. It has an effect on only part of the immune system, specifically suppressing a chemical called interleukin-2, so it does not increase the risks of infection in the way that other immunosuppressant drugs (e.g. steroids) do. There are some concerns about a possible increased risk of developing cancer after long-term treatment, so careful follow-up is usually advised even after treatment has ended. Transplant patients do have an increased risk of some cancers, but they have much larger doses of ciclosporin.

I have to have my blood pressure taken regularly because I take ciclosporin. Why is this?

Like all drugs, ciclosporin has the potential for side-effects, the main problems being possible kidney damage and high blood pressure. Both of these unwanted effects are reversible (i.e. kidney function and blood pressure will return to normal) if they are detected early, so regular monitoring is essential. We hope that you are also having regular blood tests to look at your kidney function. The blood pressure often does rise a little with this drug, but as long as your kidneys are OK you can continue with the treatment. It can be so successful that patients are reluctant to stop it, so occasionally an additional drug can be given to control the blood pressure without long-term risks.

There are a number of lesser side-effects that can be a great nuisance. These include pins and needles in the fingers, a mild tremor (shaking or trembling) and nausea, but these usually occur early in treatment and improve if it is continued. More troublesome can be extra hair growth and enlargement of the gums. The former can be particularly upsetting for women as it is not just scalp hair that grows but other body hair as well, and they may stop treatment because of it. Enlargement of the gums is more common if dental hygiene is poor so can be minimised by regular visits to the dentist.

My doctor says that taking ciclosporin can make it difficult to treat other conditions. Why is this?

Ciclosporin does interact with a number of oral treatments but not with topical ones. This interaction means that the side-effects of ciclosporin are more likely to occur, or it may not work at all. This is because the other drugs can alter enzymes in the body that affect how quickly you get rid of ciclosporin – too quickly and it will not work, too slowly and you will get many more unwanted effects. You must tell any doctor who is treating you that you are taking ciclosporin as there is a long list of problem drugs. Avoid buying over-the-counter drugs in shops where there is no pharmacist to advise you, and do not take herbal or other remedies for which the effects are unknown. The common problem drugs are:

- **antibiotics** – erythromycin (a common antibiotic) should be avoided but penicillin is safe;

- **antifungals** – itraconazole is a drug used to treat fungal and yeast infections such as ringworm or thrush;

- **painkillers** – aspirin and related drugs including ibuprofen (Advil, Brufen and Nurofen) and mefenamic acid (Ponstan) should be avoided, but paracetamol is safe;

- **antimalarials** – chloroquine can interact so avoid it if travelling abroad;

- **blood pressure tablets** – diltiazem is one to avoid;

- **tablets for epilepsy** – carbamazepine and phenytoin.

How long will I have to take ciclosporin for?

This depends on how severe your psoriasis is and how well you tolerate and respond to the drug. There are two ways to use ciclosporin – short-term/intermittent or long-term maintenance. In general, if your psoriasis is not too severe, you will be offered treatment for 4–12 weeks to try to clear your skin. Once your skin has cleared, the ciclosporin will be stopped, but you could have other short courses if it recurs. If your psoriasis is severe or keeps coming back very soon after a short course, you will probably need maintenance treatment. In this case, you could start in the same way but the dose will be reduced as your skin clears, down to the lowest dose that keeps it clear or keeps it at a level you are happy with.

Ciclosporin works well for me, but my blood pressure is a bit high so I have had to reduce the dose. My psoriasis has come back a bit, so would any of the creams help?

Using a moisturiser will always help your skin to feel more comfortable. There are good reports of using calcipotriol cream (Dovonex) with low-dose ciclosporin, so you could try this.

Other tablet treatment

I haven't had any success with methotrexate or ciclosporin. Are there any other types of tablet I could try?

There is a drug called hydroxycarbamide (it used to be called hydroxyurea) that is used in cases like yours. It does not cause any liver or kidney problems but can affect the bone marrow and hence your ability to produce new blood cells. This is thought to be more of a risk than that posed by the other drugs, so it is not used as a first choice. Treatment is usually given in courses of up to 8 weeks, but weekly blood tests are needed to check for side-effects.

I have heard that steroids can work very well in psoriasis. Can I ask my doctor to give me some?

The problem with taking steroid tablets is twofold. They have too many unwanted effects when taken by mouth, and even if they clear the psoriasis quickly, it tends to come back in a much more severe way. This tendency for psoriasis to 'rebound' after steroids is well known and can be life-threatening as the skin fails to do its job of regulating body temperature and preventing loss of fluid, so patients react as though they have had extensive burns. Paradoxically, in these severe cases, steroids can be used as a last resort but then have to be withdrawn very slowly and carefully. The only other time that steroids are used in psoriasis is when there is the added problem of psoriatic arthropathy. If the latter threatens to damage the joints irreversibly, steroids can stop the damage more quickly but will then need to be replaced by other drugs that are safer to take in the long term.

Treatments for psoriatic arthropathy

What treatment should I be having for my psoriatic arthropathy?

This depends on how badly affected you are. The aim of treatment is to improve your quality of life, deal with any inflammation in the joints and try to prevent any permanent damage to your joints. The first type of treatment to try is a non-steroidal anti-inflammatory drug (NSAID), as mentioned in Chapter 4. This may sound complicated but is in fact the first type of tablet to try in lots of different types of arthritis. One example is readily available, both on prescription and over the counter – ibuprofen (Nurofen). You might well have tried this before seeing your GP, so he or she might try different types of NSAID before referring you to a specialist.

I have joint and skin problems with my psoriasis and wonder if I should see a different specialist as well as my dermatologist.

This depends on several things. The most important is how bad your joint problems are because the worse they are, the more helpful it would be for you to see a rheumatologist – the name for a specialist in joint problems. It also depends on your dermatologist as some become expert in treating psoriatic arthropathy and can certainly start some of the second-line treatments if NSAIDs are not enough. Some hospitals have combined clinics where dermatologists and rheumatologists work together, so you would see both types of specialist at the same visit to the hospital. We feel that this is an ideal setting to help you if you have both severe psoriasis and severe arthritis, but it is not something that every hospital can provide. It would not be cost-effective to provide this type of 'super-specialist' clinic locally, but at least one should be available in every region.

**The simple treatments my GP has prescribed don't seem
to be helping my psoriatic arthropathy. What other
treatments are there?**

As with psoriasis on the skin, this is where second-line treatments
are used. Doctors talk about 'disease-modifying anti-rheumatic drugs'
(DMARDs) as this indicates that the drugs alter the disease itself
rather than dealing with the symptoms (e.g. pain) or the effects of
the disease (inflammation). These drugs are not specific to psoriatic
arthropathy but are used for many different types of arthritis:

- **Methotrexate** is also used for other types of arthritis, so it
  fits in well if you have skin and joint psoriasis. It has been
  dealt with earlier in this chapter, where the dosages and
  precautions are discussed. It is taken as a small weekly
  dose and needs careful monitoring.

- **Steroids** are powerful anti-inflammatory drugs so can have
  a dramatic effect in treating an acute flare-up of arthritis. In
  some cases, they are also used long term in low doses to try
  to keep a balance between the benefits and the potential
  side-effects listed in the section on 'Steroids' in Chapter 4.
  If steroids are used in high doses, careful monitoring of any
  psoriasis on the skin is essential because rapid changes in
  steroid dose can cause problems, with dramatic worsening
  of the skin, sometimes to the point of pustular psoriasis or
  erythroderma (discussed in Chapter 2), which are medical
  emergencies.

- **Sulfasalazine** (Salazopyrin) is being used increasingly
  often in psoriatic arthritis. It is another type of anti-
  inflammatory drug that was used mainly for inflammatory
  gut diseases such as ulcerative colitis. People with ulcerative
  colitis can get a type of arthritis affecting the lower back,
  and they noticed that this as well as their gut problems
  improved when taking sulfasalazine. It was tried in other
  forms of arthritis and does seem to work well in psoriatic
  cases. Some rheumatologists now use it as a first-choice
  tablet treatment and then add in methotrexate if needed.

- **Other agents.** Immunosuppressive drugs such as azathioprine and ciclosporin are sometimes used but seem less effective for the arthritis than they can be for the skin.

- **Gold injections** are used less often than they were in the past for all forms of arthritis. They were only rarely used for psoriatic arthropathy because one of the common side-effects is a skin rash! They worked well in a few patients so might be considered as a last resort if nothing else has worked.

- **Leflunomide** is a tablet treatment that is used mainly in rheumatoid arthritis but can be useful in some other types of arthritis. It is a DMARD.

My joints are awful and nothing seems to work. My consultant has started me on leflunomide but it doesn't seem to work either. What can I do?

If you have only recently started it, you should persevere as it can take up to 6 weeks before you notice any difference, and it could be 6 months before you get the full benefit. This can be very difficult as we know you will feel that the regular check-ups with blood pressure and blood tests to make sure your liver and blood count are OK will seem a price not worth paying yet. Stick with it though as leflunomide can give very good results in resistant cases such as yours.

My GP mentioned some new drugs given by injection. Will the specialist offer me these?

Your GP must be referring to a new class of drugs that are often referred to as biological therapies or biologics. These are designed to work in very specific parts of the chemical pathways leading to inflammation. They work right down at the level of specific cells (T-cells) by stopping them moving into the skin or by blocking the substances produced in the skin that attract the T-cells. Examples of names you might hear are etanercept, infliximab, alefacept and efalizumab – not the easiest drug names to pronounce!

They were originally used in other forms of arthritis, but their use in people with psoriatic arthropathy proved their value in treating the psoriasis itself. Several have now been licensed to treat moderate-to-severe plaque psoriasis when the individual has not responded to, or cannot take, other systemic therapy, including ciclosporin, methotrexate and PUVA. At the time of writing, the licensed ones are efalizumab, etanercept and infliximab. They all involve injections being given at a range of intervals from twice a week to once every 2 months, with a cost of £500–£1000 a month, and they can be effective for otherwise difficult-to-treat psoriasis.

Why can't I try these new treatments?

The use of these drugs is limited to those with severe disease who have tried other second-line therapies that have not worked. In addition, not all dermatologists will be using them because they may not see enough patients with severe psoriasis who are not helped by other treatments. Large departments, often linked to universities, are more likely to use new drugs and to carry out the research necessary to make sure that they are safe, effective and worth the cost. Any new treatment has to be properly evaluated in the following way:

- It should be compared with existing treatments to decide exactly where it should fit into the range of different drugs.
- Patients should be involved to help to decide whether it is an easy treatment to use and produces a real improvement in quality of life.
- It should undergo a 'health economic analysis' to make sure it is affordable and that the extra money would not help more people if spent on other drugs or treatment resources.
- It should be studied long term to try to identify all the possible side-effects.

Because these biological therapies are new to psoriasis treatment, it will take some time to determine their exact use within the National Health Service. We hope that they will be a helpful addition to the range of second-line therapies available, but they are not a 'miracle cure' and they are not suitable for everyone to use.

I have just started on methotrexate for my joints but it hasn't helped yet. Can I still take some ibuprofen?

The answer is 'Yes' – but carefully and after discussion with your specialist or your GP if he or she has experience with using methotrexate. Ibuprofen and similar NSAIDs do affect (interact with) methotrexate because they alter the way in which the body gets rid of it. This tends to raise the level of methotrexate in your body and thus increases the chance of side-effects. As you are in the early stages of treatment, you are likely to be on a low dose, so this will not be as important. Rheumatologists tend to be more relaxed than dermatologists about the two drugs being used together as they see many more patients with joint problems and have seen the benefits of improved mobility and reduced pain for their patients. Once again, it is a question of discussing your own situation with your doctor and weighing up the potential benefits against the possible risks. As you are moved on to higher doses of methotrexate, those risks will become greater, so do not assume that it will always be safe for you to take ibuprofen.

Other treatments

I have heard that lasers can be used to treat psoriasis. Is this available on the NHS?

The laser treatment of psoriasis is still being researched and evaluated so is not freely available at present. A few years ago, it looked as though it might prove successful and would become more widely available, but research has not really suggested that it is worth the investment in expensive equipment. One early approach was to remove the plaques with a laser, but this was unsuccessful. Better results seemed to come from tuning a laser to destroy the blood vessels feeding the plaques, but the more likely use of lasers may lie in treatments similar in nature to PUVA. Lasers are capable of activating chemicals applied to plaques so that they directly affect the disease process itself. As you can guess, this will still not provide a cure, but it could be a very useful alternative to

UV light treatments. Other forms of non-UV light are also being looked at, particularly a very focused red light – the equipment for this is also cheaper than a laser.

Antibiotics help with infections and were used when I first got a rash many years ago. Would they help my psoriasis now?

In general, no. The only type of psoriasis that can be helped by antibiotics is the guttate form, in which the trigger has been a throat infection caused by the *Streptococcus* bacterium. A toxin produced by the bacterium is the cause in these cases, and even if the throat seems better, it is worth taking a course of an antibiotic to ensure that the bacterium is eradicated, so no further toxin is produced to drive the psoriatic reaction. This sounds as if it was your first experience of psoriasis, so you had the right treatment at the time. Unfortunately, it sounds as though you have gone on to develop more typical plaque psoriasis, and this is not helped by antibiotic treatment. It may be a good idea for you to make sure that any sore throats you get are not caused by the *Streptococcus* bacterium as a new infection could trigger a flare-up of your psoriasis. Most sore throats are caused by viruses and do not need any antibiotic treatment, but it would be worth you getting the nurse at your doctor's surgery to take a swab from your throat to be tested for the bacterium just in case.

Using creams is so messy and time-consuming. Why can't I take pills instead?

This is a good question but one that is very difficult to answer as we do not know any details of your psoriasis. In general, creams and ointments are safer than pills because their actions can be limited to the skin. The side-effects of pills are well known to doctors, and, when deciding on the best treatment for you, they have to balance the side-effects with any possible benefits. If your psoriasis is very bad or widespread, the balance is in favour of tablets, but if the psoriasis is less widespread, it can be a very difficult decision. We feel that patients should be very much involved in making this type of decision as they are the ones 'doing' the treating.

Creams can be messy and time-consuming and have 'side-effects' on quality of life, so it is very tempting to look at different types of treatment. The daily routine of applying creams can be tedious, even with psoriasis that affects only a little of the total skin area, and sometimes people need a break. This can be achieved by using tablets or other non-cream treatments for a short while.

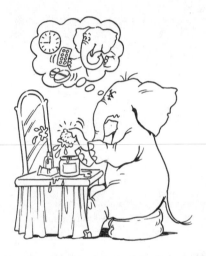

None of the simple treatments has helped my nails – what can I do to improve them?

Treating the nails is very difficult. You should keep them short to avoid further damage from catching them and have the clippings analysed to make sure that you do not have a fungal infection. A fungal infection can be an additional problem with damaged nails but can also mimic the typical changes of psoriasis. Vitamin D agents applied topically to the affected part can sometimes work if applied and covered with polythene, but this may only be practical at night. Other treatments include injecting the growing part of your nail with a steroid or using some of the tablet treatments. Nails do sometimes improve if the rest of the psoriasis clears up. If your nails are badly pitted, nail beauticians can advise you about special lacquers or fillers that are safe to use when you have psoriasis.

6
Complementary therapy

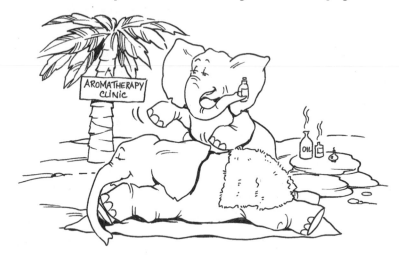

Introduction

These days, almost all health books for patients or their families need to contain a section on complementary or 'non-conventional' treatments. These used to be referred to as 'alternative', but as many of them are becoming more accepted and regulated, they are best thought of as 'complementary' to reflect the fact that they can sit alongside conventional treatments rather than replacing them. Although there is no scientific evidence that, for example, aromatherapy or reflexology is effective in treating psoriasis itself, these techniques are often very helpful in making you feel better or more relaxed.

A whole range of different approaches to helping you with your psoriasis are available outside the National Health Service (NHS), and many practitioners are genuinely trying to improve the quality of life of their clients. It is true to say, however, that there are also some people and clinics who make exaggerated claims for their particular approach or product. There is little regulation of this activity, although a report from the All Party Parliamentary Group on Skin has looked at what can or should be done to help to protect consumers by using existing Trading Standards legislation or by introducing new powers for the Medicines and Healthcare products Regulatory Agency.

There is a wealth of information available on all sorts of different ways to treat psoriasis, and we are sure that there are many new treatments awaiting discovery or proper evaluation. It is the evaluation that makes this chapter very difficult to write. People who get better from complementary treatment are always very positive about it, as are the practitioners, and you will very rarely find people advertising the fact that a treatment has failed to work or has made them worse. Most of the success stories are what we would call 'anecdotal evidence' – based on what people have reported about how they have found relief – and a lot of anecdotes are needed to make a proven case. Proper scientific studies are needed to fully evaluate different therapies and prove their safety. It may not matter whether patients choose to spend money on a treatment that does not work, but it does matter if it makes them worse or ill in some other way. Every year, we hear reports or people dying from the toxic effects of herbal remedies, both Chinese and Western, so great care is needed in choosing a complementary practitioner.

Many 'miracle cures' now seem to be advertised direct to the public. Some of these have been found to contain undeclared potent steroids, and we recommend extreme caution before you buy or use anything without first taking advice from a doctor or recognised complementary practitioner.

Choosing a safe practitioner

Most complementary practitioners work privately and are better than NHS doctors at 'selling' their treatment. They also tend to spend more time with patients, and there is an undoubted benefit in being able to talk about your psoriasis and its impact on you. It can be very relaxing to talk, and we wish the NHS system could allow more time than it does for consultations. This is not to say that the only benefit from complementary medicine comes from spending money to buy 'protected time'. It is worth remembering that the term 'complementary' is used deliberately instead of 'alternative' as these treatments should sit alongside the standard first-line treatments and not replace them.

There are now professional bodies that regulate most forms of complementary treatment, and you should contact them before choosing a practitioner. Remember that you do not need any medical qualifications to work in complementary medicine, so discuss your plans with your GP so that you can at least check whether the practitioner gets the diagnosis right.

The Royal College of Nursing has put together some very sensible guidelines for you to use when choosing a practitioner. This advice is also reflected in information produced by the Prince of Wales Foundation for Integrated Health (see Appendix 1), which also tells you much more about each type of therapy.

- What are his or her qualifications, and how long was the training?

- Is he or she a member of a recognised, registered body with a code of practice?

- Can he or she give you the name, address and telephone number of this body so you can check?

- Is the therapy available on the NHS?

- Can your GP delegate care to the practitioner?

- Does he or she keep your GP informed?

- Is this the most suitable complementary therapy for your psoriasis?

- Are the records confidential?

- What is the likely total cost of treatment?

- How many treatments will be needed?

- What insurance cover does the practitioner have if things go wrong?

Then ask yourself the following questions:

- Did the practitioner answer your questions clearly and to your satisfaction?

- Did he or she give you information to look through at your leisure?

- Did the practitioner conduct him- or herself in a professional manner?

- Were excessive claims made about the treatment?

You should avoid anyone who:

- claims to be able to cure psoriasis completely;

- advises you to stop your conventional treatment without consulting your GP;

- makes you feel uncomfortable – you need a good relationship if you are going to get full benefit from the treatment.

In short, you should demand the same standards from the practitioner as you would from a NHS doctor and subject the claims to the same critical scrutiny that is increasingly applied to NHS treatment.

Aromatherapy

Is it safe to have an aromatherapy massage with psoriasis?

Yes it is, if the massage is confined to normal skin. Massage can be very relaxing, and this can help you cope with having psoriasis. You should avoid having any large plaques massaged as the friction and oils may irritate the skin. Areas where the skin is simply dry will benefit from the moisturising effect of the oils. As with other techniques that involve touch, this in itself can be very enjoyable if you find that other people tend to recoil from touching you when they see your psoriasis.

Reflexology

What is reflexology, and can it help?

Reflexology is a massage therapy that uses acupuncture points on the feet that represent different parts of the body. The feet are massaged with talcum powder, and you do not need to take any other clothes off if you are self-conscious about your skin. Again, the contact can in itself be beneficial, and it is another good way to relax and feel more able to cope with having psoriasis. This in itself seems able to influence the disease as a positive attitude can help your body to fight it.

Chinese herbs

Chinese medicine is said to have made great advances towards helping the disease by looking at it as a whole-body problem and using herbs to adjust the balance. How dangerous is this? Will it become available on the NHS?

Chinese herbal treatments come in two main forms: creams, and preparations taken by mouth. The latter are most commonly used and have been subject to some trial work by traditional doctors. There seems to be some evidence that this treatment can be beneficial in psoriasis, but studies have been quite small scale and need further evaluation. It is unlikely that the treatment will become available on the NHS in the foreseeable future as the licensing of drugs and similar items takes many years and is very expensive. This is necessary to try to exclude any products that might have dangerous long- or short-term side-effects.

- There is no evidence that Chinese herbs cure psoriasis, but there may be some benefits.

- Chinese herbs are not always safe as they can cause inflammation of and damage to internal organs such as the liver and kidneys in the short term. The long-term side-effects are unknown.

- The raw ingredients or herbs are not under any form of quality control, so the chemical composition can vary enormously. Different countries of origin, times of year picked and storage of the herbs can all have an effect on quality.

- There is a similar lack of control over the 'doctors' who sell the herbs. They are not medically qualified Western doctors under the control of the General Medical Council. Many are responsible practitioners, but you must remember that anyone can sell these herbs. A lot of money can be made if you think that the cost can be £20–£30 per patient per week.

Recent reports ranging from undeclared potent steroids in Chinese herbal creams and deaths from kidney failure have highlighted the potential dangers of these preparations. There are calls for better regulation and more research, which are echoed by the reputable practitioners themselves. In the next few years, we may be able to recommend a range of herbal treatments, but at present we would caution against them.

Other herbal remedies

Are there any non-Chinese herbal remedies?

Yes, there is a strong tradition of Western herbal medicine with roots going back into folklore. Unfortunately, there seems to be even less published work in this area, so there is very little substance on which someone with a conventional approach can base their advice. Herbalists do spend time taking a good history and tend to use creams that can be soothing and act as a good emollient, if nothing else.

Many of our modern remedies have been produced after the study of traditional plant-based remedies, but an active ingredient needs to be identified and thoroughly tested before it can be licensed as a drug. This may well ignore the beneficial effects of groups of extracts that may, on their own, be ineffective but that work well together.

What is *Mahonia aquifolia*?

This is a plant otherwise known as the Oregon Grape. Extracts have traditionally been used to treat a variety of conditions, of which psoriasis is one. It is applied in an ointment, and some studies have suggested that it can help some patients. How it works is a mystery, but it may merit further investigation.

Other approaches

Does hypnotherapy work at all?

It may help by relaxing you and giving you a more positive approach to the disease, making it easier for you to cope with. It seems to work well if your skin is very itchy as it can help you to scratch less. Scratching an itch is often pleasurable, and you can get locked into a cycle of itching and scratching, itching and so on. Hypnotherapy can help to break this cycle and give your skin a chance to rest. We do not know of any worthwhile studies to show that it directly helps the psoriasis.

Would homeopathy help my psoriasis?

Homeopaths believe that the symptoms of a disease are actually the body's way of fighting the disease. They try to help this reaction by using minute doses of a substance that would normally produce the same symptoms if used in a higher dose on a healthy person. This 'remedy' is produced by multiple dilutions so that no more than a trace of the substance is present, and the resulting treatment is usually safe and free from side-effects. It is difficult to know whether you could benefit as psoriasis is not one of the diseases that homeopathy has been shown consistently to help. For further information, contact the British Homeopathic Association (address in Appendix 1).

A lot has been said about the Dead Sea and its benefits, and I understand that some countries such as Germany will help towards the cost of treatment there. Would it not make more sense for the NHS to pay for patients to go there rather than pay for expensive drug treatment here?

This is an attractive but rather oversimplified view. The combination of the concentrated salt solution that is the Dead Sea and strong sunshine does seem to be of benefit, but the precise mechanism has not been fully evaluated. The sea water also contains some tars, which may also be of benefit. Holidays in sunny places can be relaxing, and if other psoriatic patients are at the same resort you would be much less afraid to take your clothes off and expose your psoriasis, thus getting more benefit from the sun. As the Dead Sea is below sea level, the atmosphere is relatively thicker and does absorb some of the UVB light, which causes burning. This means that you can get a higher concentration of the helpful UVA light without burning, although this could lead to higher risks of skin cancer. Most of the reviews of Dead Sea treatment mention treatment times of under 3 hours. It is thought that the complex salt solution does add to the efficacy of natural sunlight and may in itself have some effect on skin cell turnover. However, even dermatologists from the Ben-Gurion University in Israel stress that treatment guidelines and standards have to be set in order to assess the cost-effectiveness of Dead Sea therapy, compared with other treatments.

The NHS has to be very careful about spending money, and many other patients might demand holidays because they felt better afterwards. One of the authors has asthma and it always improves on holiday, away from pollution, etc. Does this mean the NHS should pay for a holiday? Some of the philosophy behind this question is outside the scope of this book.

I saw an advert for Dead Sea mud. Could this save me the cost of a trip to Israel?

You will probably be wasting your money. In the context of the Dead Sea, the dark mud seems to help with ultraviolet absorption and can be useful as a mud pack on painful joints to help increase the circulation. This is probably not specific to the type of mud found around the Dead Sea and sold in the UK.

Dead Sea bath salts should probably be looked at in the same way. As mentioned in the previous answer, they may have a beneficial effect when combined with the UV light around the Dead Sea but on their own there is little evidence to make the product worth buying.

Is it true that special bathing pools in Turkey can cure psoriasis?

No. I think you are referring to the 'fish that treat psoriasis', as featured in the national press some years ago. There are fish in Turkish bathing pools that nibble away the plaques of psoriasis, but they certainly don't cure it! Removing the plaques does allow treatment to reach the underlying skin more easily, and this includes sunlight, so the psoriasis may well clear for a while, although it is just as likely to recur.

How can I find out more about the products advertised in the newspapers?

A very useful source of information is an American website called the 'Psoriasis Hall of Pshame'. It welcomes comments about unusual claims for treatments and reviews the latest 'scams' for you to make your own mind up about.

7
Children and psoriasis

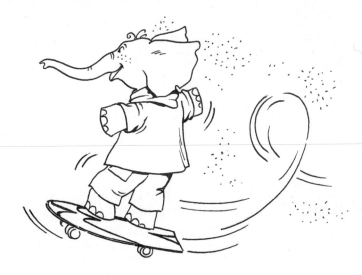

Introduction

Although psoriasis is much less common in childhood than other skin problems such as eczema, about 10% of adults with psoriasis seem to have developed it before the age of 10. If children do have it, the average age when it starts (age of onset) is 8 years, and unlike adults, for whom there is no difference between men and women, girls are more likely to have psoriasis than boys. Some studies have put this difference as high as 2:1.

There are other differences in that the rash may not appear in the same patterns as with adults, although 65% of children still have the typical distribution of large psoriatic plaques over the knees, elbows and lower back. Guttate and scalp psoriasis are more common in childhood, as is psoriasis in the napkin area and flexures (e.g. groin, armpit and behind the knee). This type of psoriasis is the most common form when infants are affected and is often mistaken for a more straightforward nappy rash.

Because children are not just small adults, the management of their psoriasis must take into account certain factors:

- Both the child and his or her parents need educating about the disease.

- The wishes of the parents and the child may be different with respect to the aims of treatment.

- The psychological effects on the child must not be overlooked, especially as other children can be brutal with teasing and bullying at school.

- There are higher risks to children from the absorption of certain creams as they have more skin surface relative to their overall size compared with adults.

- Because there is a lack of medical research into their effects on children, many treatments are actually not licensed for use in childhood. This needs to be properly discussed before parents consent to treatment for their child.

Babies and psoriasis

My baby has a bright red rash under his nappy. I have psoriasis and worry that he has it as well.

Rashes in the napkin area can be very confusing, but psoriasis is quite likely if the rash is bright red. Psoriasis does not show scales under a nappy and in the skin creases around the bottom, so it does look red and glistening. It will be very clearly demarcated – i.e. it will be very obvious where the rash stops and normal skin takes over.

My baby has psoriasis. I thought only old people got it.

Psoriasis can occur for the first time in people of any age, but your baby is unlucky as it is relatively rare in young children. It most commonly 'presents' (first appears) between the ages of 10 and 40, with some peaks at times of bodily changes such as puberty and the menopause.

Childhood infections

My 7-year-old daughter had guttate psoriasis after a throat infection. Should she have her tonsils removed?

If she has had only one attack, the answer is 'No'. There is some evidence that having their tonsils removed (tonsillectomy) does reduce the number of severe attacks of guttate psoriasis in children who get it frequently or reduces flare-ups in plaque psoriasis. On its own, however, having psoriasis is not a reason to have her tonsils taken out.

My daughter has been told that she has tinea amiantacea in her scalp. I thought 'tinea' was a medical word for ringworm – has she got this as well as psoriasis?

Your daughter does have psoriasis in the scalp, and in children the build-up of scale can be dramatic, coating the hair and causing hair loss. However, any loss will not be permanent, as the underlying psoriasis does not scar the skin or damage the hair follicles. The name is confusing and reflects the fact that the first doctors to label it felt that it was caused by ringworm; it is one of several inappropriate names for skin diseases that have persisted despite a better understanding of their cause.

Children and steroids

My daughter has a lot of psoriasis and it responds very well to steroid creams, but our GP is reluctant to prescribe them. Can I insist that he does?

Your GP is obviously well aware of the risks of using steroids in young children. All but the mildest should be avoided if at all possible, especially if a large area of skin needs treating. Children's skin allows for a much easier absorption of drugs than does adults' skin, and this is made more of a problem by the size of children. They have more skin surface area for absorption in relation to their total body size compared with adults, so greater care is needed when using creams that can act throughout the body. Steroids applied to the skin can be absorbed in high enough concentrations to have the same side-effects as though they were taken by mouth. You need to listen to your GP, and he needs to be able to offer you an alternative treatment or an opportunity to visit a hospital specialist.

Children and psoriatic arthropathy

My 4-year-old daughter has a swollen knee and one painful finger, and the consultant looking after her thinks it is because I have psoriasis. Does this mean I have caused her psoriasis?

You have absolutely nothing to feel guilty about, and we are sorry to hear that you have been worried. There are some forms of arthritis that affect young children, and one of these is called *juvenile psoriatic arthritis*. The skin form of psoriasis is uncommon in children, so the rash may not be seen for many years. The arthritis tends not to affect very many joints, is not symmetrical and can affect both small and large joints, so your daughter's seemingly odd 'presentation' with a knee and a finger affected would have suggested psoriasis as a possible cause. Because you have psoriasis, this diagnosis is more likely as your daughter has probably inherited the tendency in the same way that you did. You had no control over this!

We are glad to learn that your daughter has a consultant looking after her as this type of childhood arthritis can be quite troublesome and last longer than similar types for which there is no suspicion of psoriasis.

I have talked to other parents at the out-patient arthritis clinic that my daughter goes to, and some of them have to take their children to an eye specialist as well. Should I arrange this for my daughter?

It can be confusing talking to other parents as you probably take your daughter to a clinic for children with lots of different types of arthritis. Although the psoriatic type can be more troublesome, some of the other types may have more serious complications. One of these, called uveitis, has inflammation affecting the eyes that can cause long-term problems and even blindness – hence the need for regular eye checks. Although it occurs only rarely in psoriatic arthritis, do not feel shy about asking your daughter's consultant about this. If seeing an eye specialist is important, he or she will arrange an appointment.

School problems

The teacher says my son can't go to school. What should I do?

If your son's teacher is excluding him from school, this is a serious problem. You must talk to the teacher and head to establish exactly what the difficulty is. Your GP, the school nursing service, the local community paediatrician and your consultant will be able to help you. There are no grounds for excluding children who have psoriasis, and your school needs help to understand the disease and not be afraid of it. It is a sad fact that many people who do not know very much about skin problems react in this way as they are concerned about 'catching' the same rash.

My daughter is having swimming lessons with the school, but teachers have said they can't help her put her creams on afterwards as they have a 'no touching' policy. I don't want to tell her she can't go swimming as she really enjoys it – what can I do?

This is a very difficult question to answer. We fully appreciate the problems facing teachers as they are open to all sorts of allegations if they touch pupils. You will have to discuss this with the school governors to see whether there is a way round it. The school might have a trained first aider who might agree to apply creams, or your daughter could see whether one of her friends could help her. If the swimming session is towards the end of the school day, your daughter might be OK if she used an emollient soap substitute in the shower after swimming. This would help to stop the skin drying out too much, and she could apply her creams with you as soon as she got home.

8
Feelings, family and friends

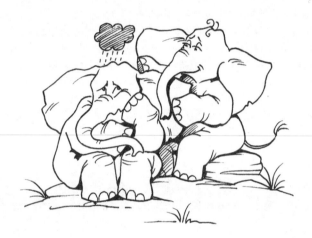

Introduction

The psychological impact of almost any disease is very important.
This is especially true for psoriasis, for which not only the
appearance of the plaques, but also the consequence of the showers
of scales that can come off need to be taken into account. Staying
at other people's homes or even trying on clothes in a shop can be
very difficult because of the fear of leaving scales behind. The effect
on each individual will vary, but not in a simple way; it is not just
linked to the severity of the disease. People will respond in different
ways, and the disease will have a whole range of impacts on
individuals' lives. There is no right and wrong way to respond, and
no one should feel guilty for experiencing very negative feelings
in relation to their psoriasis. There is, unfortunately, a lack of public

understanding of all skin diseases and a great need for more basic information about what skin looks like when it is not 'normal'. We all suffer from the impossible perfection portrayed in the media so our response to minor blemishes, never mind the response to real skin problems, can be extreme.

People with psoriasis do not live in isolation so the disease affects not only them, but also their family, loved ones and friends. The aim of the advice offered in this chapter is to encourage you to live as normal a life as possible (bearing in mind that 'normal' is different for each individual), using the help and support of those around you. Because each person and their family and friends are different, it is not always easy to give straightforward answers to questions about coping and about the feelings associated with having psoriasis. In this chapter, we offer advice that has been helpful for many of the people we have come into contact with.

Relationships

I have just met a girl I really like, but I don't want her to find out I've got psoriasis. What do other people say?

People handle these situations in different ways. We would, however, say that if you think this relationship is likely to last, you should tell your girlfriend that you have psoriasis. There are two reasons for this. First, she is likely to notice the plaques – especially if you become intimate. Second and more importantly, you will probably feel better and more relaxed once you have told her. Although it sounds like a cliché, if she really likes you, the fact that you have psoriasis will not make a difference to how she feels.

In terms of how you tell her, you can take one of two approaches. You could show her some of your affected skin and try to talk to her about psoriasis or, if you find this too difficult, you could tell her that you have psoriasis and give her some information leaflets or lend her a copy of this book. She can then read up about it herself and come back to you with questions. In general, people tend to find that they feel much better once they have told their girlfriend/boyfriend as there is then nothing to hide.

What can I do to avoid embarrassment in personal relationships?

The best way to avoid embarrassment is to be as up front as possible with your partner. By explaining what psoriasis is, you help to get round some of the awkward feelings. As we have said before, psoriasis is not your fault and does not reflect badly on you as a person. Trying to keep this in mind when you approach your personal relationships may help you to avoid embarrassment.

I have psoriasis on my penis and find it quite painful to have sex. What is the best treatment to use?

Because the skin on your penis is relatively delicate, this limits the range of treatments that you can use on it. The preferred active treatment is usually a mild topical steroid, but simply using a moisturiser may help to soothe it and lessen any scaling. Using condoms may help to protect your penis and make sex less painful. Do be aware that most condoms are damaged by oil-based substances (e.g. baby oil) and any ointments. If these substances are on your penis, the condom will not be safe. Durex, however, make a non-latex condom called Avanti, which they claim is safe for use with oil-based substances, so you should be safe with this type of condom after using ointments. Do note, however, that the condom may slip off your penis more easily during intercourse if you have applied a greasy ointment or cream prior to putting on the condom.

If you do not use condoms, applying a lubricant when having sex might make it less uncomfortable. Do not have sexual intercourse after applying any of the active treatments to your penis; they are not intended for internal use and might affect your partner badly. The other thing to bear in mind is that the friction your penis experiences during sex may aggravate the psoriasis. Refraining from having sexual intercourse until the psoriasis goes may be an option you and your partner could consider. In the meantime, of course, there are other ways of expressing loving feelings – for example, cuddling and fondling.

My wife is very hard to live with since she developed psoriasis. Can it affect a person's character?

Living with psoriasis is very distressing for some people and may, as a consequence, change the way they behave. Not only can psoriasis cause a great deal of physical discomfort, but it can also affect people's self-esteem and the way they feel about themselves. These two things together may seem to change a person's character. We suggest that you try to talk to your wife about how she feels – she may think that you feel differently towards her now that she has psoriasis, and you need to reassure her. Think about how your feelings and behaviour towards her might have changed – you might not be as intimate with her as you used to be. Touching is even more important now that she has psoriasis so you could try to help her with applying her creams. If you can feel as comfortable with her now as you did before, it should make her feel better. In a very practical sense, it is important that she gets the best treatment available; a visit to the doctor or practice nurse may be helpful to ensure that her treatment is as good as possible. Your GP might be able to refer her to a psychologist, which some people find very helpful.

Finally, talking to others with psoriasis is a good way of getting support and makes people realise that they are not alone. The Psoriasis Association has local groups that do a lot of good work, fund-raising and increasing the profile of psoriasis in society. Your local group can be contacted through the national association (address in Appendix 1). If there is not one nearby, perhaps you and your wife could start the ball rolling. Although the main focus of the Psoriatic Arthropathy Alliance (address in Appendix 1) is for people with psoriatic arthropathy, they also provide information about psoriasis.

My 25-year-old son has just developed psoriasis, and I feel so guilty about this that I can't talk to him about it. What should I do?

First of all, the guilt you are experiencing is quite commonly felt by parents when their children develop psoriasis. Although your feelings are understandable, there is no point in your blaming yourself because it is not something that you can have had any control over. Although the susceptibility to psoriasis is inherited, many people carry this gene unknowingly as they do not develop the active symptoms themselves. What is most important is that you *do* talk to your son about it. One of the things that makes coping with psoriasis easier is to have people around you who support and help you. At this potentially difficult time of his life, your son will need your understanding more than ever. If you approach him and he does not want to talk about it, it is probably best to respect this, but make sure that he knows that if he *does* want to talk, you will always be there for him.

Feeling 'different'

I feel so isolated and alone – nobody seems to understand what's happened to me.

Many people with psoriasis feel isolated and alone with their condition. The statistics, however, tell a different story: at least 1 in every 50 people has psoriasis – think how many people at your average football match must have it! Isolation often occurs because people feel unable to talk to others about their psoriasis, especially when it has first been diagnosed. The most effective way of getting round the feelings of isolation is to seek support from others around you. Although you may feel embarrassed to talk about psoriasis, others will not be able to help or support you unless you do and thus let them know how you are feeling. Support groups are good places to find help: the people there understand what you are going through as it is likely that they will have had similar experiences themselves. Addresses of possible support groups are given in Appendix 1.

My psoriasis is ruining my life. Everything I try to do seems to be affected by the state of my skin and I can't look forward to anything. How can I change this?

Your story is only too familiar. Psoriasis can rule your life. To break free and change the way it affects you, you may need the help of a psychologist; your GP or consultant should be able to refer you to one. People often cope with psoriasis by avoiding situations that might cause embarrassment from other people's comments. Examples include not accepting invitations to stay with family or friends for fear of leaving scales on the floor, and not exposing your skin to the sun even though it would probably help. A psychologist will work with you to change the way you feel about yourself and your skin.

Psychologists cannot change the fact that you have psoriasis, but they can influence the way you think about it. As well as this, they teach relaxation techniques and interpersonal and social skills. You should end up feeling much more confident in yourself as a person, with a degree of control over your psoriasis so that it no longer dominates your life.

I get so irate when people say to me 'it's only skin', as if having psoriasis is not a serious problem.

It is true that many members of the public do not understand the serious impact that psoriasis can have on people's lives. Because psoriasis is rarely life-threatening and the skin is seen as not that important, they do not appreciate the severe physical and psychological discomfort that it can cause. What you can do in these situations is try to explain how it feels to you having psoriasis and also point out how important the skin is as an organ of the body. For example, the skin is the largest organ of the body and is responsible for protection, temperature regulation, sensing pleasure and pain, defence mechanisms through the immune system and, of course, our appearance. All you need to do is look at the beauty industry to see how important the appearance of the skin is! Ask people if they would say 'it's only skin' if all the bits of your skin affected by psoriasis were burned? The next time someone makes an insensitive comment about its 'only being skin', be ready with your response so that they are left in no doubt about the important role that the skin has to play in health and well-being!

I feel like it is all my fault that I have got psoriasis, and blame myself for letting it wreck my life.

It is quite common for people to blame themselves for having psoriasis, but let's look at the facts. There is no doubt that, to have psoriasis, you need to have the gene or genes that make you susceptible to it. You could not have done anything about this. To show active signs of psoriasis, this gene needs to be activated or triggered. These trigger factors have been discussed in Chapter 3. Most people at some point in their life experience one or more of these trigger factors, and they will respond to them in different ways. For you, your body responds by developing psoriasis; this is not your fault, and you should not blame yourself for it. The aim of this book and of the various support groups that exist is to help people to make sure that having psoriasis does not wreck their lives. The hope is that, by highlighting ways of managing it both physically and psychologically, people will feel better able to live life to the full and make the most of it.

A lot of people say that stress is what causes psoriasis. I always feel as if they are suggesting that I don't cope well with stress when in fact I think I am quite a calm and 'together' person. What do you think?

There is little doubt that stress is one of the potential trigger factors for psoriasis. However, the point you are making is one commonly reflected by others with psoriasis – they get fed up with people saying it is stress that causes psoriasis and insinuating that the individual must be unable to cope with the stress in their life or else they would not have developed the condition. Although the evidence does point to stress having an effect on the development of psoriasis, this does not automatically mean that you are bad at coping with it. We all experience difficult situations in our lives, and although the experience of stress is affected by our

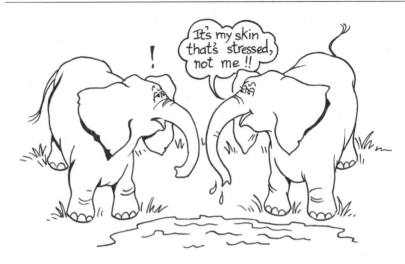

psychological state, it is also a physiological response that happens automatically in our bodies and over which we have little control. As with most things in psoriasis, this is very individual: some people are absolutely certain that experiencing stress makes their psoriasis worse; others do not see such a direct link. Lumping everyone together and making generalisations is not helpful and not especially accurate.

Feeling embarrassed

I get so embarrassed when I go out because I can't help scratching.

Psoriasis can be very itchy indeed, and it is difficult to stop yourself scratching – people often find that they do it subconsciously without even noticing. Because of this, it is helpful to keep your fingernails short so that, if you *do* scratch, you cause less damage. Once you start scratching, although you might get relief at first, it often makes you feel itchier in the long run. Stopping scratching can therefore make you feel less itchy.

Your skin is less likely to be itchy if your treatment is effective. Moisturising in particular is very helpful because it is cooling and soothing, and you can apply lots of it. Rather than scratching, try applying some moisturiser. The principles of moisturising apply to your scalp as well as to your body – massaging coconut oil into the scalp acts as an excellent moisturiser.

Other helpful tips to minimise the likelihood of your scratching while you are out include wearing cool, loose-fitting cotton clothing and avoiding sitting close to direct sources of heat. If you can be aware of what your hands are doing (e.g. folding them on the table), this can reduce the temptation to scratch. Some people use a 'counter' that they click each time they want to scratch; this just increases your awareness of the desire to scratch and can decrease your scratching dramatically. Finally, if you are with close friends or family, it might be worth asking them to tell you when you are scratching so that you can stop before you really get going.

I sometimes get a bit of psoriasis on my face and I am very aware of people looking at it when I am talking to them rather than focusing on what I am saying. What can I do?

People will always look at blemishes on someone's face – one's eyes are so often drawn towards a spot or a patch of psoriasis. It is quite unnerving, though, when you are trying to get a serious message across, to feel that they are not concentrating on what you are saying. Really the only solution, other than ploughing on regardless of the stares, is to try to make the patch of psoriasis less obvious by applying lots of moisturiser and by using a cover-up make-up. This last suggestion is easier for women to follow, but the British Red Cross and the British Association of Skin Camouflage (addresses in Appendix 1) offer a very effective camouflage service (for both men and women) using special techniques to cover up unwanted skin changes.

If you know the person you are speaking to, you may feel comfortable enough to tell them that you have psoriasis and mention that they seem to be staring. This tactic is harder if you are talking to a stranger, but why not try it – you might be pleasantly surprised by their response. The charity Changing Faces, mentioned in Appendix 1, has done a lot of work with people embarrassed by their appearance. One of the key ways of coping is to make, and keep, eye contact with the person you are speaking to. They soon start to feel uncomfortable about their initial reaction to you.

Feeling fed up

The treatments that I have been given to do are so time-consuming and expensive that I feel like just giving up and living with the psoriasis.

This is a decision that you are, of course, free to take. It is your skin, and if you feel able to cope with it not using any treatment, that is absolutely fine. Before you take this decision, however, it is probably worth considering three points. First, have you and your doctor explored all the possible options for treatment – are you perhaps just fed up because you do not have a treatment that fits in with your lifestyle? Second, have you explored all the options for getting cheaper prescriptions (see Chapter 10) if cost is a real problem? And, third, if you stop doing anything, your psoriasis may get worse.

If you do decide to stop treating your skin with any active treatments, it would be very wise to continue moisturising. Choose a nice light lotion, which can be very quick to apply and will have a minimal impact on your life but will help to keep the psoriasis less dry and therefore more comfortable.

My doctor is too busy with people who have problems more serious than mine to keep bothering her about different treatments.

It might sometimes seem this way, but it is important that you feel able to see your GP whenever you need to discuss the treatments you are using and whether or not they are working. Your GP is there to provide care to *all* the patients on her books, and she will not think that you are any less important than the other people she sees. We keep mentioning the importance of the skin – it is the largest organ in the body and is very important. Look around the waiting room and try to guess what everyone else is bringing to their GP.

Many of them will have seemingly minor and often self-limiting illness but will need, and value, the GP's care and reassurance. If, however, you feel that you are not getting the information you need about the treatments from your GP, you might like to ask whether there is anyone else who can help – there may be a nurse available who has more time to discuss things with you. It may also be worth considering making contact with the Psoriatic Arthropathy Alliance or the Psoriasis Association. Both organisations have access to information about treatments as well as being support groups for people with psoriasis who may be experiencing the same sort of thing as you.

9
Lifestyle and looks

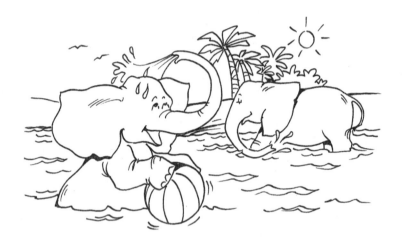

Introduction

Any glance at a magazine rack in a shop will show the number of publications for men and women dealing with lifestyle and looks. In this chapter, we hope to provide answers that can help you to avoid problems in achieving the look you want, and in living life the way you want. This is not always easy. People with psoriasis are well known for buying patterned carpets because these help to disguise the shed scales!

These days, many diseases are judged by the impact they have on quality of life, and studies have shown that psoriasis is up there with heart disease in terms of the problems it can cause. In one study, people unlucky enough to have both diabetes and psoriasis were more likely to choose psoriasis if offered the imaginary chance of a cure for one of their diseases. All health-care workers should ask patients with psoriasis about the impact of the disease on areas such as holidays, work, sport and their sex life. People will often not bother the doctor with what they consider are trivial questions, but they are probably the most important issues to deal with if life with psoriasis is to be as normal as possible.

Clothes

What are the best types of clothes and materials to wear?

The short answer is 'Whatever feels most comfortable to you.' Smooth fabrics that do not rub or aggravate plaques (e.g. soft cotton or silk) are probably the best. Creases or seams can sometimes be uncomfortable if they rub psoriasis so they are best avoided – likewise, tight trousers might worsen any plaques on your legs. Scales from your psoriasis will not show up as much on light-coloured clothes as they do on darker ones so this may be worth considering. If you are applying very messy, greasy treatments, you will find it easier to have a set of clothes (e.g. shirt and track suit) that you put on while the treatment sinks in.

My psoriasis seems to be worse where my clothes rub, for example round my waist. Why is this?

The 'Koebner phenomenon' is the medical term for what you have described. Psoriasis can get worse in areas where the skin is rubbed or damaged in any way. So, for example, where you fall over and cut yourself, psoriasis is more likely to form in the scar; or if you have an operation, psoriasis is more likely to form along the line where the surgical cut was made. Also, if you constantly scratch or pick your psoriasis, this is also likely to make it worse. Note that there is not a 100% link – psoriasis will not always form at the point of injury – but it significantly increases the likelihood. The skin does not have to be broken to cause the Koebner phenomenon, as this question demonstrates: it can occur where constant rubbing is present.

My washing machine gets ruined by all the grease that I have to use as part of my treatments. Can you make any suggestion for how to prolong the life of my machine?

The grease in the heavier-duty moisturisers (the ointments) causes the rubber seal around the washing machine door to disintegrate. There is, as yet, no total solution to this, but manufacturer Hotpoint suggests that the rubber seals can be made to last longer by periodically doing an empty wash at 35 degrees Celsius (95 degrees Fahrenheit) with biological powder. (This presumably dissolves the grease and makes it less likely to damage the rubber.) Writing to washing machine manufacturers about this problem will ensure that they know it is a real problem for users – and hopefully encourage them to develop more durable rubber seals!

There are a couple of other practical measures you can take that might help to prolong the life of your machine. First, if you have garments that are heavily impregnated with grease, soak them in a bowl of very hot water with some washing detergent or, perhaps better, soda crystals – this will help to remove some of the grease. The second possibility is to change your moisturiser to one that is less greasy. This will obviously depend on how severe your psoriasis is, but it may be possible to use a less greasy moisturiser more often and still keep your skin adequately moisturised. If it is the active treatment that is making your garments greasy, you might consider asking your doctor to prescribe you the cream rather than the ointment form. Although creams tend to be less good than ointments at keeping your skin moisturised, they are more acceptable cosmetically.

Staining

Clothes and soft furnishing get very stained with the treatments. Can you suggest ways of preventing this or of removing the marks?

Once soft furnishings have been stained, it is generally difficult to remove the stains. If it is possible to hot-wash them, this may get rid of grease stains, but tar and Dithrocream tend to stay put. If you get tar or Dithrocream on the floor or furniture, remove it with a cloth as quickly as possible (this limits the staining).

The best course of action, therefore, is prevention and, failing that, 'damage limitation'. If you are using tar or Dithrocream at home, make sure that you have some sets of clothes that you wear after the treatment; this way you ruin only a limited number of garments. Always try to do your treatment in one place – probably the bathroom – and stand on old towels to protect the flooring. When you have finished doing the treatment, use old towels to protect the furnishings. If you are doing a scalp treatment, try to do it before bed and go to bed with the treatment on, protecting your pillows with two or three old pillowcases.

Another possible course of action is to ask your doctor whether you could change to a less messy treatment option; this may not always be appropriate, though. You might also like to ask for some tubular cotton bandages (e.g. Tubifast), which can be used to help keep the treatment in place and stop it getting rubbed off.

Cosmetics and personal appearance

Can I wear make-up when I have got psoriasis?

There is no reason why you cannot wear make-up. If you have psoriasis on your face that you want to cover up with make-up, do a small test area first to make sure that the make-up does not aggravate it. Be sure to remove any make-up at the end of the day and then apply plenty of moisturiser.

My 12-year-old wants to get her ears pierced. Will this make her psoriasis worse?

If she is careful and uses an experienced piercer rather than doing it herself or letting a friend do it, she should have no problems. There are, however, some risks. She might develop psoriasis at the site of piercing (the Koebner phenomenon) or, if she developed an infection, this might cause a general flare-up. Having her ears

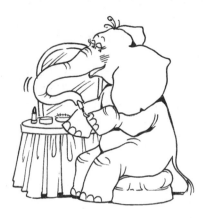

pierced is, however, part of being normal despite the psoriasis, so we would suggest that you allow her to go ahead.

Can I wear nail polish?

Yes, nail polish is fine for you to use. Be a bit careful with nail polish remover because, if you have sore fingertips, this will make them sting.

My nails are pitted so nail varnish looks rough – is there anything I can do about this?

You can get an acrylic filler to apply to your nails to smooth out any pits or other irregularities before applying varnish. The best way to find out more about this is from a nail beautician.

Will dyeing my hair do the psoriasis in my scalp any harm?

When considering dyeing your hair, the thing to be careful about is worsening the scalp psoriasis by applying astringent chemicals to it. Bleaching the hair, for example, would probably make scalp psoriasis worse. Hair dyes are much less aggressive than they used to be, and you may well be able to find one that suits. However, our advice is that you do not try tinting or colouring your hair at home but instead take advice from your hairdresser, who should have the most up-to-date information about possible options. Hairdressers are taught about skin conditions that affect the scalp and should be knowledgeable enough to offer advice.

Many people feel embarrassed about going to the hairdressers, but a good hairdresser will not shy away from doing your hair. If you feel concerned about going to the hairdressers, why not try phoning first and explaining your situation to one of the stylists? If they sound sympathetic over the phone, you can book to see them and you will not have to feel you need to do any explaining once you are there.

Quite large lumps of my hair have come out. Is this normal?

It is quite usual for hair to fall out when psoriasis is active in your scalp. When you descale your scalp, you may find that your hair particularly seems to fall out – especially when the plaques are treated or when you comb or brush your hair. Although it is worrying to see your hair come out, it will grow back once the scalp psoriasis has been successfully treated as psoriasis does not cause long-term damage to the skin and does not affect the hair follicles. It can take several months for the hair to grow back.

Can I remove hair from my legs?

Yes, you can. But if you shave and cut yourself, this might lead to new patches of psoriasis appearing (the Koebner phenomenon, discussed earlier). Also note that plaques of psoriasis tend to bleed more easily than other skin so waxing or sugaring your legs might cause pinprick bleeding (i.e. little specks of blood across the surface of the plaque).

Applying treatments seems to make the psoriasis look worse. Is this true, and if so, why?

This does seem to be the case for many people. Applying ointments or creams to your skin gets rid of the scaliness on top of the plaques, which then emphasises the redness of the plaque underneath. This particularly seems to be the case if a greasy ointment is used. If you are rubbing the ointments into the plaques, this can cause the blood vessels to dilate so that the blood comes to the surface of the skin, thus increasing the red appearance.

You can do two things to minimise the impact this has on you. First, if you find that the treatment makes your psoriasis look redder, try to apply it with sufficient time for the redness to die down before you go out. Second, apply the treatment gently (although you do need to rub it in). Do not, whatever you do, stop the treatments: although they might make the plaque look temporarily worse, they are doing a good job and will show good results in the long run.

I have quite dark skin, and I find that after I clear the plaques of psoriasis I am left with patches of lighter skin. Is there anything I can do about this?

It does seem that, on clearing the psoriasis, people are sometimes left with areas of skin that are lighter than the rest of their skin; this will be particularly obvious if you have dark skin. These areas will eventually 'recover', and the normal pigmentation will return – but it may take up to a year. This phenomenon occurs in all skin types but is more noticeable in dark or tanned skin. The reverse sometimes happens too in skin that is already quite dark or pigmented; for example, people of Asian or African origin can go even darker once the skin problem has cleared.

Swimming

Will it hurt or worsen if I go swimming?

No – swimming itself does not harm your psoriasis. If you swim in a chlorinated swimming pool (as opposed to the sea or a lake), the chlorine can, however, have a drying effect on your skin. Making sure that you wash your skin very thoroughly following your swim and applying plenty of moisturiser before you get dressed can counteract this.

You may find that some people will stare or make unpleasant comments when you go swimming, but most will probably take very little notice. You should not be asked to leave the pool by the authorities, but you might feel more comfortable approaching the pool manager before getting into the pool, just to check that he or she is not going to object. It is important to tell people that psoriasis is not catching; sometimes they can be ignorant about what psoriasis is, which makes them react in a negative way. It could be worth taking some information literature with you to give to anyone who asks you, which will save you having to explain yourself. You can photocopy Appendix 4, which has the basic facts for you to pass on.

Some support groups arrange special sessions at a pool so that there is more than one person with psoriasis there, or they may arrange a session specifically for people with psoriasis. In any case, try to be confident: remember that you have as much right to swim and enjoy yourself as anyone else.

I'd rather die than feel noticeable. What can I do to avoid embarrassment on the beach or in the swimming pool?

The embarrassment is often caused by wondering what other people are thinking about your psoriasis. There are two ways of coping with this. First, ignore the odd glance that you may get – people are generally a lot less interested than you think they are. We are all 'guilty' of looking at people around us to see what they are wearing, how they look in a swimsuit, etc. – it is no more than a passing interest. Second, confront people in a polite but firm way, especially if you feel that they really are staring at you. Try to make – and keep – eye contact with them to stop them looking at your skin rather than you! Have ready prepared in your head a little spiel that you come out with, for example, 'I have a skin condition called psoriasis. It is quite common. It makes my skin grow too fast . . . and don't worry, because you can't catch it.' Most people will accept this sort of explanation.

As mentioned in the answer above, you have as much right as anyone else to swim or lie on the beach. It is not your fault that you have psoriasis, and it does not make you any less of a good person. The embarrassment is something you feel in yourself – use the support of your friends and family to help you get over it. Take them with you when you go swimming so that you do not feel so vulnerable or isolated. Most of all, enjoy yourself and try not to focus on what you think other people are thinking about you.

Other considerations

Should I give up smoking?

Yes, you should give up smoking – the health benefits of doing so are significant for everyone. Some research suggests that smokers are twice as likely as non-smokers to develop psoriasis. Smoking is bad for your skin in general, as it speeds up the ageing process. So, although stopping smoking will probably not make your psoriasis go away, it might help to contribute to it not coming back again, and it will certainly have a very positive effect on your overall health as well as on the quality of your skin.

Would it help if I emigrated?

There is little doubt that sunny weather helps to control psoriasis for many people so, for them, living in a sunny climate might well help. Sunshine is not, however, helpful for everyone, and some find that it worsens their condition. If you were to seriously think about emigrating, you should also give consideration to the health services available in the country you hope to go to. In some countries (e.g. South Africa, New Zealand and the USA), you might not have access to a public health service so the cost of private health care needs to be carefully considered. It is also worth remembering that psoriasis is not as common in some parts of the world so you might feel even more uncomfortable about having it.

Would it help if I lost weight?

If you are definitely overweight, losing weight will not do you any harm and will indeed significantly benefit your overall health and well-being. It is unlikely, however, to have a direct effect on your

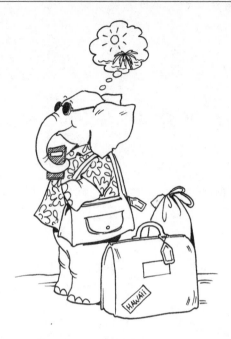

psoriasis. Having said this, being overweight can give you extra folds of fat, which produce deep creases in which you can develop psoriasis. These areas can be difficult to treat so losing weight can make life easier in terms of being able to do treatments. If the fact that you are overweight gives you concern and makes you feel less good about yourself, resolving this might help to put you in a better frame of mind to cope with and manage your psoriasis.

If I had a large patch of psoriasis taken off and a skin graft done, would it stay away forever?

No, it would not stay away. Psoriasis develops because of changes occurring in the immune system. These changes would affect a new skin graft in the same way that they affect your old skin: the skin used for a graft is taken from a different part of your body; it is not like a 'transplant' from somebody else. This means that you would have a damaged area from where the graft was taken that would be likely to develop psoriasis (the Koebner phenomenon).

10
Practical concerns

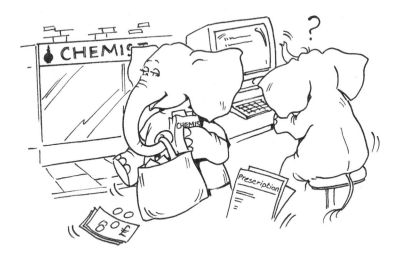

Introduction

In this chapter, we try to answer the many questions that people ask about the financial and other practical aspects of living with psoriasis, including what is happening in medical research.

Money questions

Is there any way of reducing the cost of prescription charges if I have to have several items a month?

Yes. If you are one of the minority in the United Kingdom who pay for prescriptions, you can lessen the burden by obtaining a prepayment certificate. Your GP or pharmacist should have details about how to obtain this from the Prescription Pricing Authority, using form FP95 (EP95 in Scotland). Alternatively, you can go online and purchase one directly at Prescription Pricing Authority website or buy one with a credit card over the phone (contact details in Appendix 1). The price is linked to the cost of prescriptions so it can change when prescription charges are altered, but if you have more than five items in 3 months or more than 14 in a year, it is well worth doing. Certificates can cover a quarter or a full year.

It is also worth checking whether you are exempt from prescription charges. You can find out from a leaflet entitled *Help with Health Cost?* (HC11), available from post offices, Social Security offices and NHS hospitals. In general, people who do not have to pay for prescriptions are:

- people aged 60 or over;

- people aged under 16;

- people aged 16, 17 and 18 who are in full-time education;

- people (and their adult dependants) receiving Income Support, income-based JobSeeker's Allowance, Pension Credit or Guarantee Credit, and those with an NHS Tax Credit Exemption Certificate;

- women who are pregnant or have a baby under 12 months old;

- people with certain medical conditions (psoriasis *not* being one of them).

Note: This list is correct at the time of writing, but you can be sure with such lists that the contents will vary. Consult your GP, pharmacy or the local Citizens Advice Bureau for the latest information.

Some of the treatments that are used for psoriasis are available over the counter (without a prescription). Buying them this way is sometimes cheaper than getting a prescription. Do note, however, that it sometimes works the other way round, something obtained with a prescription being cheaper than buying it over the counter.

The tables in Appendix 3 will give you some idea of comparative costs, although clearly prices do change.

If you live in Wales, your prescription charges will be less than in England and Scotland and free up to the age of 25. It is anticipated that prescriptions will be free to everyone by 2007, but this depends on changes agreed in Parliament and might be affected by elections!

My husband has very bad psoriasis and the arthritis that goes with it. I am unable to work as I have to care for him, and we have very little money. Are there any benefits we could claim?

Yes, at least two come to mind. Your husband could be eligible for Disability Living Allowance (DLA). This is not means-tested so any savings or other income he has should not affect it. The DLA is based on the amount of care needed and varies depending on your husband's individual needs. It also has a component for mobility, and this could mean that he is eligible for a vehicle through a contract hire scheme organised by Motability (address in Appendix 1).

If your husband gets the DLA, you may be entitled to claim Carer's Allowance for yourself: you would have to be spending 35 hours or more a week caring for him. This benefit is also not means-tested but does have to be declared for tax purposes. Further information is available from any Benefits Agency office or from the Benefit Enquiry Line (see Appendix 1), requesting form DS700. The government website (again see Appendix 1) gives a lot of useful information about living with disability, including further details of benefits that might be available to you and your husband.

Jobs

Are there any jobs that I cannot apply for because I have got psoriasis?

You can apply for any job that you want – the response you receive to your application will depend largely on the current state of your psoriasis and how bad it has been in the past. Many employers will have very little interest in the fact that you have psoriasis, particularly if it has not had an adverse effect on your previous employment record. There are, however, some employers – including the armed forces – who are more likely to question you about your psoriasis and perhaps even reject you because of it: one of the armed forces' exclusion criteria is widespread psoriasis. It is important to note that this is not a blanket approach, and their ideas are often out of date; if you have a real passion for doing a specific job, you should apply for it on the assumption that individual assessments need to be made.

On a personal level, it is important for you to think through the impact of your psoriasis on any job you might do. If, for example, you have very bad psoriasis on your hands and/or under your fingernails, this might make doing a job that involves fine movements with your fingers difficult and painful. If you are the right person for a job, a good employer should help you to find ways of coping with your psoriasis at work so that it has a minimum impact on your comfort and what you do. Occupational health departments in the workplace are often helpful sources of information and support. Jobcentres have disability advisers who may be able to provide information about jobs and benefits that you might be eligible for.

The future

What hopes are there for a cure in the future?

A cure for psoriasis may be possible at some point in the future, but this is unlikely to happen in the next few years. Current research suggests that there is more than one gene linked to psoriasis – possibly as many as 16 or more – which in turn suggests that there are a number of different types of psoriasis. Research on this issue may lead to the development of new treatments that are better targeted to the specific type of psoriasis. In the future, it is thus likely that increasingly effective treatments will be developed, which will make managing the disease less of a problem and will

make life easier. New therapies are now being licensed in Europe
that will mean an increased range of options for those with severe
psoriasis in the future. These new therapies, known as biologics,
are given by injection. It is too early to assess what sort of impact
they will have on individuals with psoriasis in Great Britain, but
this marks a major development in the treatment of psoriasis. (For
further details on biologics, see Chapter 5.)

Is there much research being done?

There is research going on in a number of different areas:

- genetic research to identify the gene (or genes) that causes
  (or cause) people to develop psoriasis;

- exploration of the immune system – especially
  T-lymphocytes (a type of white cell), which are thought
  to have a major contributory effect on the development
  of psoriasis: manipulation of the immune system may
  eventually provide us with some 'cures' for psoriasis;

- looking for different and better treatments for psoriasis in
  terms of developing new creams, ointments and tablets;

- the effect that psoriasis has on people's lives. The
  information gained helps health-care professionals to have
  a better understanding of the impact of psoriasis and helps
  to improve dermatology services. This research is also used
  to improve the public's awareness and understanding of
  psoriasis;

- looking at the way in which different individuals respond to
  different external stimuli such as stress and infection, and
  at how this affects their psoriasis.

There are many different institutions and organisations
undertaking research. The Psoriasis Association uses a significant
proportion of its funds to provide money to health-care
professionals and scientists so that they can carry out research
into all sorts of different areas related to psoriasis. If you want to
find out more about this research, visit the Psoriasis Association

website (see Appendix 1). If you are interested in being a volunteer for a research project, patients' organisations often have information about current research projects that are recruiting patients. Your local dermatology department may also be looking for volunteers for research that it is doing.

I have been asked to take part in a research study as a volunteer. Should I agree to do this?

The decision of whether or not to get involved is entirely up to you, and you should feel under no obligation to take part in a research study. If, however, you are keen to help out, there are some things that you should think about:

- Have you been provided with crystal-clear information about what the study will entail?

- Have any risks or potential side-effects been explained to you?

- Have you been told that you can withdraw at any point?

- How will your privacy be protected?

- How will you find out about the results of the study?

It is worth mentioning that, by taking part in a well-designed study, you are helping to progress the development of the understanding of psoriasis and possible treatments for it. We cannot, however, overemphasise the importance of your feeling content that you have received adequate answers to the questions listed above and any more you may have.

Will there be a genetic treatment in the future to fix faulty genes?

This is highly unlikely. Better genetic understanding will help to design better treatments, but as psoriasis is linked to many different genes, fixing one gene would not help even if it were possible.

More help and information

My GP does not seem to know or care. How can I get to see a specialist?

There are two ways that you can get to see a skin specialist (dermatologist): either through your GP or by paying to see one privately. If your GP refuses to refer you to a dermatologist, you could ask to talk to another GP to see whether he or she is of the same opinion, but it is definitely worth discussing with your GP why he or she does not think you need referral to a specialist. The National Institute for Health and Clinical Excellence (NICE; see Appendix 1) has published guidelines for GPs about when patients should be referred to specialists so it might be worth looking at these before any discussion.

You are, of course, free to change GP if you want to, and you could look for one who has a special interest in, and therefore more knowledge of, dermatology. If you decide that you want to see someone privately, you may be able to do this yourself by contacting a dermatologist directly. More often than not, though, you will still need a letter from your GP referring you to a specialist even if you go privately. Make sure that you know how much it is going to cost before you make a private appointment.

My GP says I do not need to go to hospital but I think I do, and I don't like using the steroids he gives me.

It is quite difficult if you fundamentally disagree with your GP about the care he is offering you. The best way to tackle this is to be prepared next time you go to see him. Take a list of questions asking why he is prescribing the treatment he is and requesting a trial of something else. Topical steroids are sometimes helpful for some types of psoriasis, but they are not generally considered to be the best long-term treatment, so you are right to think about asking for an alternative. If you feel that you need hospital treatment, you should ask your GP to explain why he believes that hospital treatment is inappropriate. You can ask to talk to another GP in the practice to see if he or she has an alternative opinion.

I sometimes feel so confused about how to apply my treatments. I know my GP is too busy to spend much time explaining these to me. Is there anyone else who might be able to help?

It is quite understandable that you might feel a bit confused about which treatments to use when and how to apply them. This sort of support is what specialist nurses who have a specific interest in skin disease can offer. Some GP practices employ a nurse with this sort of expertise so that they can improve the care offered to people with skin disease, including psoriasis. The nurse should have more time to explain to you how to use your treatments and may arrange for you to see him or her on a regular basis to assess how you are getting on. There is a general move to try to limit the demand placed on hospitals by making more specialist treatment and management available in the community. You could contact your MP to make sure that this will include skin problems in the area where you live.

  You may also find that your pharmacist can be a very useful source of advice – especially if you always take your prescription to the same one.

How can I find out about the most recent treatments available?

Your GP will have some information about recent treatments but is unlikely to be aware of everything that is available. The Psoriasis Association is a very good source of information, and its newsletter (distributed to all members four times a year) often contains reviews about new treatments on the market. Your local hospital dermatology department is likely to have information about the latest treatments, but it is not always easy to get this information unless you have an appointment with the department. If you have access to the Internet, the British Association of Dermatologists' website (address in Appendix 1) provides a lot of information. The Psoriatic Arthropathy Alliance offers excellent information through newsletters and a journal, as well as a CD-ROM. It also holds an annual conference, which has useful presentations, exhibits, discussions, etc. NICE, mentioned earlier, also publishes information on some areas of treatment; for psoriasis, this includes the newest treatments.

At a recent meeting I heard other people with psoriasis talking about dermatology specialist nurses. Would it be helpful for me to see one, and how can I find out if there is one working in my area?

Dermatology specialist nurses are qualified nurses who have chosen to specialise in the field of dermatology and as such have a lot of knowledge and skills relating to skin problems. They are particularly good at helping people to make the most of their treatments, and at providing psychological and social support to those who are struggling to cope. Many people find it very helpful to see this sort of professional, and we have little doubt that it would be helpful for you too. Dermatology specialist nurses are not, however, always easy to find. If you receive hospital care, there are likely to be specialists in the department, and it is worth asking what they can offer. As mentioned above, there are an increasing number of specialist nurses working in the community with GPs so it is worth asking next time you see your doctor. One final message on this point is that there are more and more nurses gaining skills in dermatology, particularly in primary care, so although your local community nurse (e.g. practice nurse or district nurse) may not be a specialist, she or he may well be able to help you.

Where can I get more information about psoriasis?

Appendix 1 of this book includes organisations and sources of information that you can use to find out more. There are an increasing number of addresses available on the Internet. Putting the word 'psoriasis' into a 'search engine' will find a number of these, but Appendix 1 contains some we have checked out.

Glossary

Terms in *italic* in the definitions below are also defined in this Glossary.

acute   Short-lasting. In medical terms, this usually means lasting for days rather than weeks or months. (See also *chronic*)

adrenal glands   Important glands in the body that produce a number of *hormones* to control the body systems. Cortisol and cortisone are two very important examples, and adrenaline is another.

allergy   To have an allergy means to overreact to something in a harmful way when you come into contact with it. If you have an allergy to grass pollen, you will have streaming eyes and nose and sneezing if you come into contact with it (hayfever). Someone who is not allergic to grass pollen will not even notice when they have come into contact with it.

anaemia   This means a reduction in the amount of the oxygen-carrying pigment, haemoglobin, in the blood.

anecdotal evidence   Reports from people about their experience of *triggers*, treatments, etc. – rather than scientific evidence obtained from strictly regulated tests.

antibody   A special kind of blood protein made in response to a particular *antigen*, which is designed to attack the antigen.

antigen   Any substance that the body regards as foreign or potentially dangerous.

arthritis   Inflammation of one or more joints, characterised by swelling, heat, redness of overlying skin, pain and restriction of movement.

atrophy   Wasting away of a body tissue. With skin, this means thinning and loss of strength.

barrier cream   A cream or ointment used to protect the skin against irritants.

biopsy The process of obtaining a sample of tissue (e.g. liver or skin) for analysis under a microscope.

bone marrow The tissue contained in the internal cavities of bones that is involved in making blood cells.

chronic In strictly medical terms, chronic means long-lasting or persistent. Many people use the word 'chronic' incorrectly to mean severe or extreme. (See also *acute*)

cytotoxic Something that can damage cells.

dermatology The medical speciality concerned with the diagnosis and treatment of skin disease.

dermis The deep layer of the skin.

diagnostic Something that is 'diagnostic' is a characteristic feature; it occurs so often in a disease that you do not need any other clues to know what the disease is.

distribution The pattern of a disease on the skin, for example all over, on the hands, in the *flexures*, etc.

eczema A red, itchy inflammation of the skin, sometimes with blisters and weeping.

emollient An agent that soothes and softens the skin; also known as a moisturiser.

emulsifying ointment A thick, greasy *emollient*.

epidermis The outer layer of the skin.

erythroderma An abnormal reddening, flaking and thickening of the skin, affecting a wide area of the body.

extensor The side of a limb on which lie the muscles that straighten the limb (e.g. the back of the arm and the front of the leg).

flexures The areas where the limbs bend, bringing two skin surfaces close together (e.g. the creases at the front of the elbows, the back of the knees and the groin).

genes 'Units' of inheritance that make up an individual's characteristics. Half are inherited from each parent.

genetic To do with *genes*.

guttate A term used to describe lesions on the skin that are shaped like drops of water.

hormone A substance that is produced in a gland in one part of the body and is carried in the bloodstream to work in other parts of the body.

immune system The body's defence system against outside 'attackers', whether they are infections, injuries or agents that are recognised as 'foreign' (e.g. a transplanted organ). The immune system fights off infection and produces *antibodies* that will protect against future attack.

immunity   Resistance to specific disease(s) because of *antibodies* produced by the body's *immune system*.

immunosuppressive   A drug that reduces the body's resistance to infection and other foreign bodies by suppressing the immune reaction.

in-patient therapy   Treatment carried out when a patient is admitted to hospital.

incidence   The number of new cases of an illness arising in a population over a given time.

inflammation   The reaction of the body to an injury, infection or disease. It will generally protect the body against the spread of injury or infection, but it may become *chronic*, when it tends to damage the body rather than protect it.

interleukin-2   One of a group of special proteins that control the immune response. Interleukin-2 stimulates the T-*lymphocytes* that are active in the skin.

keratinocytes   Types of cells that make up over 95% of the *epidermis* (outer layer of the skin).

Koebner phenomenon   This describes a reaction in the skin that occurs in psoriasis and some other skin diseases, in which typical lesions of the disease appear in areas of skin damaged by injury such as a scratch, cut or burn.

liver biopsy   See *biopsy*.

lymphocytes   White blood cells that are involved in *immunity*.

malnutrition   The condition resulting from an improper balance between what is eaten and what the body needs.

moisturiser   See *emollient*.

natural history   The normal course of a disease; the way it develops over time.

non-steroidal anti-inflammatory drugs (NSAIDs)   A group of drugs that act to reduce inflammation in the body, particularly in rheumatic diseases.

papular   A pattern of rash that consists of small raised spots on the skin that are less than 5 mm across.

photosensitiser   Any agent, *topical* or *systemic*, that acts to increase the sensitivity of the skin to light.

phototherapy   Treatment with light – usually ultraviolet (UV) light.

placebo   A medicine that is ineffective but may help to relieve a
condition because the patient has faith in its powers. New drugs are
tested against placebos to make sure that they have a true active
benefit in addition to the 'placebo response'.

plaque   A raised patch on the skin that is more than 2 cm across.

psoriasis   A *chronic* inflammatory skin disease.

psychologist   A specialist who studies behaviour and its related
mental processes.

pustule   A small pus-containing blister.

sebaceous glands   Glands in the skin that produce an oily substance
– sebum.

seborrhoeic   Related to excessive secretion of sebum. (See also
sebaceous glands)

seborrhoeic eczema   A form of eczema that affects the face, scalp,
upper back and chest. It characteristically produces yellowish,
greasy scales.

spondyloarthritis   A term used to describe arthritis of the spine.

steroids   A particular group of chemicals, which includes very
important *hormones*, produced naturally by the body, as well as
many drugs used for a wide range of medical purposes. In psoriasis,
the subgroup of steroids with which we are concerned is the
corticosteroids. This term is very often shortened to 'steroids',
causing people to confuse their skin treatments with the anabolic
steroids used for body-building.

subcutaneous   Beneath the skin.

systemic   This term is used for a drug, given by mouth or injection,
that affects the whole body.

teratogenic   Something that damages an unborn child.

topical   A term used to describe drugs that are applied to the skin
rather than being taken internally.

triggers   Factors that may bring on psoriasis but do not cause
psoriasis.

Appendix 1

Useful addresses

Please note that website addresses change quite frequently and quickly become out of date.

Patient support organisations

Psoriatic Arthropathy Alliance
PO Box 111
St Albans
Hertfordshire AL2 3JQ
Tel: 0870 770 3212
Fax: 0870 770 3213
Email: info@thePAA.org
Website: www.ThePaa.org
Offers useful information and support about various aspects of psoriasis, focusing especially on arthritis.

Psoriasis Association
Milton House
7 Milton Street
Northampton NN2 7JG
Tel: 0845 676 0076 (local rates)
Fax: 01604 792894
Email:
mail@psoriasis.demon.co.uk
Website:
www.psoriasis-association.org.uk
Offers useful information and support about various aspects of psoriasis.

Skin Care Campaign
Hill House
Highgate Hill
London N19 5NA
Tel: 020 7561 8248
Website: www.skincarecampaign.org
An alliance of patient groups, health professionals and other organisations concerned with skin care. It campaigns for a better deal for people with a wide variety of skin problems.

Skinship
Plascow Cottage
Kirkgunzeon
Dumfries DG2 8JT
Tel: 01387 760567
*Provides a helpline for people
with any skin disease.*

*Other useful sources
of information*

**All Party Parliamentary
Group on Skin**
26 Cadogan Street
London SW1X 0JP
Tel: 020 7591 4833
Fax: 020 7591 4831
*An all-party group specialising
in skin, which was established
in 1993 to raise awareness in
Parliament of skin disease.*

**Association of the British
Pharmaceutical Industry**
12 Whitehall
London SW1A 2DY
Tel: 020 7930 3477
Fax: 020 7747 1411
Email: abpi@abpi.org.uk
*Brings together companies in
Britain producing prescription
medicines, other organisations
involved in pharmaceutical
research and development, and
those with an interest in the
pharmaceutical industry in
the UK.*

Benefit Enquiry Line
Room 901
Victoria House
Ormskirk Road
Preston
Lancashire PR1 2QP
Tel: 0800 88 22 00
Fax: 01772 238953
Website: www.dwp.gov.uk;
see also www.direct.gov.uk
*State benefits information line
for sick or disabled people and
their carers.*

**British Association of
Dermatologists (BAD)/
British Dermatological
Nursing Group (BDNG)**
4 Fitzroy Square
London W1T 5HQ
Tel: 020 7383 0266
Fax: 020 7388 5263
Email: admin@bad.org.uk
Website: www.bad.org.uk
            www.bdng.org.uk
*Professional organisations
representing doctors and nurses
who have an interest in and/or
work directly in dermatology.
Among other things, they
provide patient information
leaflets about various skin
diseases, including psoriasis.*

**British Association
of Skin Camouflage**
PO Box 202
Macclesfield
Cheshire SK11 6FP
Tel: 01625 871129
Email: info@skin-camouflage.net
Website: www.skin-camouflage.net
*A network of practitioners
trained in camouflage
techniques for skin conditions
and disfiguring injuries.*

**British Homeopathic
Association**
29 Park Street West
Luton
Bedfordshire LU1 3BE
Tel: 0870 4443950
Website: www.trusthomeopathy.org
*To promote homeopathy and
encourage understanding and
use by the public while
campaigning for more
homeopathy on the NHS.*

British Red Cross Society
44 Moorfields
London EC2Y 9AL
Tel: 0870 170 7000
Website: www.redcross.org.uk
*Offers a camouflage service
using special techniques to cover
up unwanted skin changes.*

Changing Faces
The Squire Centre
33–37 University Street
London WC1E 6JN
Tel: 0845 4500 275
Fax: 0845 4500 276
Email: info@changingfaces.org.uk
Website: www.changingfaces.org.uk

Citizens Advice Bureau
*For a wide range of advice,
including financial and state
benefits. Look in the telephone
directory for your local branch.*

**Institute for
Complementary Medicine**
PO Box 194
London SE16 7QZ
Tel: 020 7237 5165 (weekdays
10am–2pm)
Fax: 020 7237 5175
Website: www.i-c-m.org.uk
*Information and advice about
complementary therapy.*

Long-Term Medical Conditions Alliance
Unit 212
16 Baldwins Gardens
London EC1N 7RJ
Tel: 020 7813 3637
Fax: 020 7813 3640
Email: info@lmca.org.uk
Website: www.lmca.org.uk
Made up of over 100 organisations, the Alliance campaigns on behalf of people with long-term medical conditions. Psoriasis is represented.

Motability Operations
City Gate House
22 Southwark Bridge Road
London SE1 9HB
Tel: 0845 456 4566
Fax: 020 7928 1818
Website: www.motability.co.uk
Advice and help about cars, scooters and wheelchairs for people with disabilities.

National Institute for Health and Clinical Excellence (NICE)
Website: www.nice.org.uk

NHS Direct
0845 4647
A 24-hour helpline, manned by nurses, for information about health.

Prescription Pricing Authority
Tel: 0845 850 0030
Website: www.ppa.org

Primary Care Dermatology Society
Gable House
40 High Street
Rickmansworth
Hertfordshire WD3 1ER
Tel: 01923 711678
Email: pcds@pcds.org.uk
An organisation made up of GPs who have a special interest in dermatology.

Prince of Wales Foundation for Integrated Health
Website: www.fihealth.org.uk
Provides information about integrating complementary and conventional health care.

Skin Treatment and Research Trust (START)
Chelsea and Westminster Hospital
369 Fulham Road
London SW10 9NH
Tel: 020 8746 8174
Primarily a laboratory research establishment, not an information service, but they may be able to give information about specific research questions.

Society of Homoeopaths
11 Brookfield
Duncan Close
Moulton Park
Norhampton NN3 6WL
Tel: 0845 450 6611
Fax: 0845 450 6622
Email: info@homeopathy-soh.org
Website: www.homeopathy-soh.com
Professional organisation for homeopaths, but offers a service of finding a homeopath in your area.

Additional websites

Here are some additional websites that we think are worth looking at. There are hundreds of websites available, some of which offer personal comments from sufferers and others that offer 'cures' for psoriasis. Do watch out for websites that make unrealistic claims, especially if they are asking you to part with money!

www.psoriasis.org
This is the website of the American National Psoriasis Foundation (NPF). It is regularly updated and has a lot of very good information about research and practical advice. Do note that it is American so some of the information about products may not be relevant in Britain.

www.nlm.nih.gov/medline/psoriasis
A source of very up-to-date information from the National Library of Medicine in the USA. The same warning applies as for the NPF website: some of the products mentioned may not be relevant in Britain.

www.skincarephysicians.com
A website written by American dermatologists for patients; as above, the website is based on an American health-care system and talks about American products.

www.skincell.org/psoriasis_uk.shtml
www.psoriasis-help.org.uk
Both of these are primarily forums or chat rooms for people with psoriasis. Information about the condition is also provided, but it is hard to see who has written the information and therefore to guarantee its accuracy.

www.pinch.com/skin/pshame/
An American website which tries to identify and expose psoriasis treatment scams.

Appendix 2

Useful publications

Publications for people with psoriasis

Coping with Psoriasis, by Ronald Marks, published by Sheldon, London (1997).

Psoriasis: A Patient's Guide, 3rd edn, by N.J. Lowe, published by Martin Dunitz, London (2003).

Publications for health care professionals

ABC of Dermatology, 4th edn, edited by P.K. Buxton, published by BMJ Books, London (2003).

Clinical Dermatology, by J.A.A. Hunter, J.A. Savin and M.V. Dahl, published by Blackwell Scientific Publications, Oxford (1990).

Common Skin Diseases by T.F. Poyner, published by Blackwell Science, Oxford (2000).

Dermatology Nursing, edited by E. Hughes and J. Van Onselen, published by Churchill Livingstone, Edinburgh (2001).

Handbook of Psoriasis, 3rd edn, by C. Camisa, published by Blackwell Publishing, Massachusetts (2004).

Mosby's Color Atlas and Text of Dermatology, by R. Graham-Brown and J.F. Bourke, published by Mosby, London (1998).

Nursing Care of the Skin, edited by R. Penzer, published by Butterworth Heinemann, Oxford (2002).

Appendix 3

Tables of products and their relative cost if bought over the counter

Table 1 Emollients

Name of product	Greasiness	Amount	Approx. cost 2006/7
Aveeno cream	Slightly greasy	100 ml	£6.35
Balneum bath oil	Slightly greasy	200 ml	£4.92
Dermol 500 lotion	Slightly greasy	500 ml	£11.97
Diprobase cream	Slightly greasy	500 g	£10.83
Diprobath bath additive	Slightly greasy	500 ml	£12.29
E45 emollient bath oil	Slightly greasy	500 ml	£7.36
E45 emollient wash cream	Slightly greasy	250 ml	£4.62
E45 cream	Slightly greasy	500 g	£9.89
E45 lotion	Hardly greasy	500 ml	£5.45
Epaderm ointment	Very greasy	500 g	£10.67
Oilatum emollient bath additive	Slightly greasy	250 ml	£4.85
Oilatum shower emollient	Hardly greasy	150 g	£10.22
Unguentum M cream	Very greasy	500 g	£18.70
Doublebase	Slightly greasy	500 g	£10.73
Hydromol ointment	Very greasy	500 g	£7.96

This is only a small sample of the bath oils creams, lotions and ointments available over the counter. Make sure you are using the one that suits you best and is most effective on your skin. Your doctor will prescribe most of these, and it is generally cheaper to get them on prescription – especially if you ask for the larger sizes. You may be able to get bigger or smaller versions than shown here.

139

Table 2 Tar-based treatments

Name of product	Amount	Approx. cost 2006/7
Alphosyl 2 in 1 shampoo	250 ml	£5.69
Capasal shampoo	250 ml	£7.69
Clinitar cream	100 g	£19.40
Cocois scalp ointment	100 g	£17
Exorex lotion	250 ml	£30
Polytar liquid (shampoo)	250 ml	£4
T-Gel (shampoo)	250 ml	£7

Table 3 Topical steroids classified by potency

Group strength	Chemical (generic) name	Trade name
Very potent	0.05% clobetasol propionate	Dermovate
	0.3% diflucortolone valerate	Nerisone Forte
Potent	0.1% betamethasone valerate	Betnovate
	0.025% fluocinolone acetonide	Synalar
	0.1% mometasone furoate	Elocon*
	0.05% fluticasone propionate	Cutivate*
Moderately potent	0.025% betamethasone valerate	1/4 Betnovate (otherwise known as Betnovate RD)
	0.00625% fluocinolone acetonide	Synalar 1 in 4
	0.05% clobetasone butyrate	Eumovate
	0.05% alclometasone dipropionate	Modrasone
Mild	2.5% hydrocortisone	Efcortelan
	1% hydrocortisone	Dioderm

* For use only once a day.

Appendix 4

Fact sheet on psoriasis

Here are some of the important facts about psoriasis. Please feel free to photocopy this sheet and use it to inform those around you.

1. Around 2% of the UK population (1 in 50 people) have psoriasis.
2. It affects men and women equally.
3. It is **not** contagious.
4. It is **not** related to poor hygiene.
5. It is thought to be passed on from one generation to another, but it is possible to carry the psoriasis gene without having any signs of the disease.
6. There are several factors that are thought to trigger episodes of active psoriasis:
   - Injury to the skin – for example, a cut or graze or even rubbing from clothes – may cause psoriasis to appear at the point of the injury.
   - Shock or long-term stress can cause psoriasis to develop.
   - Certain drugs are related to the appearance of psoriasis; these include beta-blockers, antimalarial drugs and lithium.
   - Drinking too much alcohol can aggravate psoriasis and will certainly make it feel worse.
   - Smoking is thought to make psoriasis worse, especially pustular psoriasis on the hands and feet.
7. People who get psoriasis can have periods of remission when they have no psoriasis on their skin at all.

8. Psoriasis is usually treated using creams and ointments, but in severe cases drugs might be taken by mouth.

9. Many people with psoriasis find that sunlight makes their psoriasis better, but 10% find that it actually makes it worse.

10. Psoriasis can feel extremely uncomfortable (dry, itchy, sore and sometimes painful).

11. Up to 15% of people who suffer from psoriasis have some form of arthritis that is specifically linked to their psoriasis.

The Psoriasis Association

Charity number 257414

- Founded in 1968 by Dr Dick Coles and a group of patients at Northampton, the Association has become an important self-help organisation providing support and mutual aid for sufferers.

- It is advised by an eminent Medical and Research Committee, and each year supports important research projects.

- Considerable publicity and education has increased the community understanding and acceptance of psoriasis.

- The Association continually works to raise standards of patient care through its contacts with the medical professions, the social services, government departments and other organisations.

- The Association has become the main source of information on all aspects of psoriasis.

- Close links have been formed with similar organisations throughout the world.

- The Association is managed by an elected Council of voluntary members supported by a small number of full-time employees.

- Membership is open to anyone. Every Member receives the national Journal *Psoriasis* three times a year. This includes articles by both sufferers and medical experts on all aspects of psoriasis.

Members may also participate voluntarily in the activities of their local Groups. These meet regularly to provide points of social contact and information, and to raise funds for research and educational projects.

Aims

To help people with psoriasis by

- Collecting funds for and promoting research.
- Advancing education in all aspects of the condition.
- Increasing public acceptance and understanding.
- Representing their national and local interests.
- Providing a point of social contact.

For contact details, see Appendix 1, earlier.

The Psoriatic Arthropathy Alliance

Charity number 1051169

The Psoriatic Arthropathy Alliance (PAA) is a national registered charity dedicated to raising awareness and helping people with psoriatic arthritis and its associated skin disorder psoriasis.

The organisation was co-founded by David and Julie Chandler (David has the condition) in April 1993, both being spurred on by the lack of adequate information available to patients and the general public.

Although psoriatic arthritis is considered by many to be a minority illness of the 2–3% of the UK population who have psoriasis, between 10 and 20% of these people will develop psoriatic arthritis, which makes it the second most common rheumatic arthritis in the UK.

Since the charity's launch in the Jubilee Room at the House of Commons, hosted by David Congdon, former chairman of the All Party Parliamentary Group on Skin, the PAA has continually achieved the following:

- Consistently produced publications for its members and professionals.
- Held annual national conferences.
- Developed its own Internet site.
- Undertaken a national awareness campaign with a spring 'awareness' week.
- Dealt with, on average, over 5,000 enquiries each year.
- Contributed to the debate for better healthcare for patients.
- Made links with similar organisations nationally and internationally.
- Developed a strong board of medical and non-medical advisers.

Membership is available to all and includes free back issues of all publications, information sheets, free entry to the annual conference and unique access to contacts throughout the UK.

For further information about the PAA or its activities, see the contact details in Appendix 1, earlier.

Index

Have you found **Psoriasis – the 'at your fingertips' guide** useful and practical? If so, you may be interested in other books from Class Publishing.

Acne – Answers at your fingertips £17.99
Dr Tim Mitchell and Alison Dudley
Acne is the most common chronic skin condition of adolescents, affecting to some extent almost all teenage boys and girls. It tends to begin at puberty, and while for most people it tends to go away by the time they reach their mid-20s, some people may continue to have acne until they reach their 40s or 50s.
> 'By far the best book I have read on the subject.'
> *Peter Lapsley, Chief Executive, Skin Care Campaign*

Eczema – Answers at your fingertips £14.99
Dr Tim Mitchell and Alison Hepplewhite
With answers to hundreds of questions on every aspect of living with eczema, this book will help you find ways to manage your own eczema – or that of your child – to fit in with everyday interests and activities.
> 'What a joy to have a new book which is medically accurate, wide ranging and practical in its approach.'
> *Margaret Cox, Chief Executive, National Eczema Society*

Gout – Answers at your fingertips £17.99
*Professor Rodney Grahame,
Dr H Anne Simonds
and Dr Elizabeth Carrey*
This is an invaluable reference guide for people suffering from gout. It offers positive, practical advice on dealing with the condition, information on the causes of gout, and advice on the beset ways to treat it and reduce chronic symptoms.
> 'It is excellent as an information resource for patients and doctors.'
> *Dr Michael L Snaith, University of Sheffield*

Arthritis £14.99
Dr John Marcus Thompson
The new, British edition of an internationally best-selling book provides clear, practical and up-to-date information on arthritis. The author covers all the most common types of arthritis as well as many uncommon types so you can identify your arthritis and manage it effectively.
> 'Up-to-date, accurate and comprehensive, telling readers what they need to know.'
> *Professor Harry Seftel,
> Emeritus Professor of Medicine,
> University of Witwatersrand,
> South Africa*

Allergies – Answers at your fingertips £17.99
Dr Joanne Clough
This new edition of a sensible, practical guide on allergies from an experienced medical expert, gives you clear and concise information on allergies – what they are, how they develop and, most importantly, how to deal with them.
> 'Excellent first-hand guidance.'
> *Professor Stephen Holgate, Southampton General Hospital*

Beating Depression £17.99
*Dr Stefan Cembrowicz
and Dr Dorcas Kingham*
Depression is one of most common illnesses in the world – affecting up to one in four people at some time in their lives. *Beating Depression* shows sufferers and their families that they are not alone, and offers tried and tested techniques for overcoming depression.
> 'All you need to know about depression, presented in a clear, concise and readable way.'
> *Ann Dawson,
> World Health Organization*

PRIORITY ORDER FORM

Cut out or photocopy this form and send it (post free in the UK) to:

Class Publishing
FREEPOST 16705
Macmillan Distribution
Basingstoke　　　　　　　　　**Tel: 01256 302 699**
RG21 6ZZ　　　　　　　　　　 **Fax: 01256 812 558**

Please send me urgently *(tick boxes below)*	*Post included* *price per copy (UK only)*

☐ **Psoriasis – Answers at your fingertips**　　　　　　　　£20.99
　 (ISBN 10: 1 85959 117 5 / ISBN 13: 978 1 85959 117 8

☐ **Eczema – Answers at your fingertips**　　　　　　　　　£17.99
　 (ISBN 10: 1 85959 125 6 / ISBN 13: 978 1 85959 125 3)

☐ **Acne – Answers at your fingertips**　　　　　　　　　　£20.99
　 (ISBN 10: 1 85959 073 X / ISBN 13: 978 1 85959 073 7)

☐ **Allergies – Answers at your fingertips**　　　　　　　　£20.99
　 (ISBN 10: 1 85959 147 7 / ISBN 13: 978 1 85959 147 5)

☐ **Gout – Answers at your fingertips**　　　　　　　　　　£20.99
　 (ISBN 10: 1 85959 067 5 / ISBN 13: 978 1 85959 067 6)

☐ **Arthritis**　　　　　　　　　　　　　　　　　　　　　£17.99
　 (ISBN 10: 1 85959 106 X / ISBN 13: 978 1 85959 106 2)

☐ **Beating Depression**　　　　　　　　　　　　　　　　£20.99
　 (ISBN 10: 1 85959 150 7 / ISBN 13: 978 1 85959 150 5)

　　　　　　　　　　　　　　　　　　　　　TOTAL _____

Easy ways to pay

Cheque: I enclose a cheque payable to Class Publishing for £ _____

Credit card: Please debit my　☐ Mastercard　☐ Visa　☐ Amex

Number _____ Expiry date _____

Name _____

My address for delivery is _____

_____

Town _____ County _____ Postcode _____

Telephone number (*in case of query*) _____

Credit card billing address if different from above _____

_____

Town _____ County _____ Postcode _____

Class Publishing's guarantee: remember that if, for any reason, you are not satisfied with these books, we will refund all your money, without any questions asked. Prices and VAT rates may be altered for reasons beyond our control.